REAL HEALTH IS SIMPLE

Forget the Noise. Simple, Lasting Principles for Real Health

LEVI MILE

Table of Contents

Introduction: The Truth About Health

If you're holding this book, you've almost certainly been overwhelmed by health advice. Some of it comes through glossy magazine covers, some through podcasts or YouTube channels, and a lot through the endless scroll of social media. Eat this, avoid that. Try this supplement, but never that one. Keto is the secret, no wait, it's intermittent fasting. Someone swears that red wine is a health food; another headline warns it's dangerous.

The messages don't just conflict, they arrive with conviction. Each new voice insists it has *the* truth, and each one implies that if you don't follow, you're falling behind. It's exhausting. A typical day in this environment might look like this: you wake up and scroll your phone. A wellness influencer recommends celery juice "to reset your gut." At lunch, you overhear a coworker talking about how carbs are "toxic." By dinner, you're watching a documentary that claims sugar is poison—or, depending on the documentary, that meat is the real culprit.

It's no wonder so many people feel like health is slipping further away as they try to grasp it.

The Paradox of Too Much Knowledge

Here's the strange reality: **we live in the most informed generation in history, yet also one of the most confused when it comes to health.**

Why? Because information doesn't equal clarity.

Science itself is complex, nuanced, and ever evolving. A single study rarely proves anything; it adds one piece to a larger puzzle. Yet, the way this research gets translated into the public sphere often strips away nuance. Headlines are designed to grab attention, not to capture complexity. "Coffee Causes Cancer" makes for clicks. "Coffee May, in

Certain Quantities, Influence Risk Factors Differently Depending on Genetics and Lifestyle" doesn't. Add in corporate marketing and social media algorithms, and the result is not education, but confusion.

And yet—beneath the noise, **something steady has always been there.**

What We Actually Know

Look across cultures, time periods, and high-quality research, and certain themes consistently appear.

- People who eat a diet rich in minimally processed foods—fruits, vegetables, legumes, whole grains, healthy fats, and moderate amounts of protein—tend to live longer, healthier lives.
- People who move their bodies regularly—not necessarily with formal "exercise" but through walking, lifting, bending, and daily physical labor—tend to maintain mobility and vitality longer.
- People who sleep adequately, around 7–9 hours depending on the individual, function with more clarity, energy, and resilience.
- People who manage stress—through practices like prayer, meditation, social connection, journaling, or even simply spending time in nature—are less vulnerable to chronic illness and burnout.
- And people who have strong relationships, family ties, friendships, and community tend to thrive in both body and mind, no matter their income or geography.

These aren't radical discoveries. They're patterns that have shown up again and again, whether in "Blue Zones" where longevity clusters, or in large-scale epidemiological studies, or even in anthropological records of traditional cultures. The irony is that we already *know* the basics. The hard part is living them in a world that sells distraction and shortcuts.

Why We Chase Complexity

If health is so simple, why do we complicate it? There are a few reasons:

1. **The allure of novelty.** We are wired to be drawn to the new and shiny. A promise of a "revolutionary" diet or "groundbreaking" discovery will always feel more exciting than "eat vegetables, sleep, and move."
2. **The business of health.** Simplicity doesn't sell well. A billion-dollar industry thrives on keeping people uncertain, offering products and programs to fill that gap.
3. **The psychology of control.** Complicated systems, paradoxically, give us a sense of control. Following a detailed diet plan or rigid protocol can feel empowering—even if the benefits aren't better than a simpler approach.
4. **The culture of performance.** In modern life, we've been taught to optimize everything: work, productivity, even leisure. Health becomes another arena where we measure and compare.

But the truth is, complexity often hides the basics. And when we lose sight of the basics, we spin in circles.

What This Book Will Do (and Won't Do)

This is not a prescriptive manual. I won't tell you to cut out entire food groups, buy exotic supplements, or adhere to strict daily rituals. If that's what you came for, you'll be disappointed.

What this book *will* do is offer a framework. Not a checklist, but a lens. A way of seeing health that makes it less overwhelming and more actionable. You'll learn how to simplify nutrition without falling into extremes, how to approach movement in ways that fit your lifestyle, how to treat sleep as the foundation it truly is, how to manage stress without shame, and how to think critically when health advice starts to spiral.

You'll also notice a specific language here: "may support," "some evidence suggests," "can help." That's intentional. I won't pretend certainty where it doesn't exist. Science evolves. Bodies differ. What works for one person might not work for another. Honesty about uncertainty is part of respecting you.

A Note on Safety & Responsibility

This book is not medical advice. I am not your doctor. I am not your therapist. The principles here are based on research, experience, and patterns, but they are not substitutes for professional care. If you have chronic conditions, are pregnant, are taking medications, or have unique health concerns, consult a qualified healthcare provider before making significant changes. This is not just legal language, it's practical wisdom. Even "healthy" practices can backfire if applied without context.

Think of this book as a compass, not a prescription. It can point you toward north, but you must decide how to travel—and sometimes, you may need a guide along the way.

Why It's Simpler Than You Think

Here's the heart of it: real health is not about memorizing endless rules. It's not about hacking biology with expensive powders. It's not about chasing what worked for someone else. It's about applying a few enduring principles consistently, in ways that fit *your* life. Eat mostly real food. Move most days. Sleep enough. Manage your stress in healthy ways. Connect with people. Keep your environment as supportive as you can.

When you do these things—not perfectly, not obsessively, but consistently—you align with what human bodies are designed for. That's when health feels less like a project and more like a rhythm.

The Invitation Ahead

The chapters ahead will walk you through the core pillars of this rhythm. You'll learn not just what the science says, but how to apply it without getting stuck in perfectionism or guilt. You'll see examples from daily life, hear about common pitfalls, and be encouraged to adapt rather than copy.

The end goal is not to turn you into someone new. It's to help you return to what your body already knows: that health is not found in complexity, but in simplicity lived with care.

This book is your toolkit for clarity. But the tools only matter if you use them. So, bring your curiosity. Bring your skepticism. Bring your real, every day, imperfect life. That's exactly where health belongs.

The journey starts now.

Redefining Health in a Noisy World

If you've ever felt overwhelmed by health advice—eat this, don't eat that, walk 10,000 steps, avoid carbs, take these supplements, meditate daily, lift heavy, stretch more—you're not alone. The modern health space has become a cacophony of conflicting voices. One moment, butter is bad: the next, it's superfood. Some swear by raw food, others by fasting, others still by cutting out entire food groups. Social media feeds us bite-sized slogans packaged as solutions, and before we know it, we've started to believe that being healthy is only for the obsessively disciplined or the well-funded.

This confusion isn't your fault. It's the result of a health culture that has become overrun by marketing, extremes, and complexity disguised as expertise. But here's the truth: real health, the kind that supports a long, functional, joyful life, is far simpler than we've been led to believe.

Redefining health starts by clearing the noise and remembering what it means to be well in the first place.

What "Real Health" Actually Means

Most of us think of health as the absence of disease. But that's a limited view. Real health is about function. It's how well your body, mind, and energy systems operate—how you feel, move, rest, focus, and recover. It's about waking up with clarity instead of fog, digestion that works quietly in the background, moods that don't swing wildly, energy that carries you through the day, and resilience that helps you bounce back from stress, colds, or the unexpected.

In simple terms, real health is your **baseline**—your ability to live and adapt well in your environment. It's not about perfection, strict regimes, or being the fittest person in the room. It's about your system working in sync, in a way that supports your goals, your values, and your everyday life. This kind of health doesn't necessarily look like magazine covers or influencer posts. It may not always be visible from the outside. Real health isn't about appearance, it's about capacity. Can your body do what you ask of it? Can your mind focus and rest? Can you respond to stress without breaking down? These are the deeper questions we should be asking.

What's empowering is that this version of health doesn't require exotic solutions. It thrives on fundamental things we already have access to, if we know where to look and how to return to them.

The Core Pillars of Well-Being

Rather than chasing the next trend or tool, it helps to ground ourselves in the time-tested foundations that human health is built upon. Think of these as the pillars holding up a structure. When one weakens, the whole system can tilt—but when they're balanced, everything works better.

These core pillars include **how you nourish your body**, **how you move**, **how you sleep**, **how you manage stress**, and **the environment you live in**. While every individual has different needs, these areas influence almost every process in the body—immune function, hormonal balance, metabolism, brain health, and more.

Let's break that down—not as a checklist, but as a framework. Nutrition isn't just about calories or rules; it's about the quality and rhythm of what you eat. Movement doesn't mean chasing athletic performance; it means keeping your body engaged, mobile, and capable. Sleep isn't just about avoiding fatigue—it's when your body does most of its repair work. Stress isn't an enemy, but how we relate to it shapes everything from blood pressure to digestion to immunity. And our environments—what we touch, breathe, absorb, and even think—can support or sabotage our well-being in subtle but powerful ways.

None of these pillars exists in isolation. When you improve one, others often follow. For instance, sleeping better can lead to better food choices.

Moving regularly can reduce anxiety. Eating nutrient-dense food can improve focus. These are not isolated acts; they're parts of a feedback loop. That's what makes health both dynamic and manageable.

The challenge, then, isn't in understanding these pillars. It's in staying connected to them despite the noise that tries to convince us we need something more extreme, expensive, or trendy to "finally" be healthy.

Why Complexity Creates Confusion (And Keeps Us Stuck)

There's an old saying: if something isn't working, complicate it. It's often said as a joke, but in the world of health, it's all too real. Overcomplication sells. It creates dependency. When people feel like health is beyond their grasp unless they follow a niche protocol or hire a specialist, they stop trusting themselves.

Think of how many "programs" exist today that offer life-changing health in exchange for strict adherence, expensive supplements, or a subscription. These systems may offer structure, but often at the expense of sustainability. Once the program ends, many people feel lost, either burnt out or frustrated.

This is not to say that expert guidance is bad, or that learning more is wrong. But when we lose sight of the basics—when we stop trusting our ability to make simple, consistent choices—we become passive consumers of health rather than active participants.

The irony is that the human body has evolved for adaptability, not perfection. We are designed to work with rhythm and feedback, not rigid control. Complexity hides that truth. It gives the illusion of progress while creating fear of failure. It replaces habits with hacks, and deep understanding with surface-level knowledge.

True health comes not from mastering a complex system but from returning to what's essential—and doing it consistently. It's not always glamorous, and it won't always be easy, but it's infinitely more empowering.

The Cost of Missing the Basics

When we get distracted by surface-level solutions, we miss opportunities to improve what really matters. Consider the person who buys a premium fitness tracker but still sleeps four hours a night. Or someone who takes expensive supplements but eats in a rush and lives in a state of constant stress. Or the person obsessed with detox products, but spends most of their day sitting, inside, under artificial light.

These scenarios are not uncommon. In fact, they've become normalized. But they highlight a pattern: we chase upgrades before we've built a foundation. And when that foundation is weak, nothing truly sticks.

The good news? The basics work. Slowly, yes—but powerfully. When we eat foods our bodies recognize, move in ways our joints and hearts appreciate, sleep deeply, and give our nervous systems time to regulate, we often find that many "issues" begin to soften. Maybe it will not disappear entirely, but become manageable, integrated into a life that supports us instead of fighting us.

Reconnecting with Common Sense

You don't need a degree in physiology to improve your health. In fact, many of the best practices are grounded in common sense: eat food that looks like food, move your body regularly, sleep when you're tired, breathe deeply when stressed, and spend time in natural light. These principles aren't hidden in labs; they've been lived by healthy humans for generations.

The challenge isn't access—it's attention. Our modern world pulls us away from this common sense. We sit more, rush more, scroll more, and sleep less. We've normalized patterns that don't support us and then wonder why we feel exhausted, foggy, or stuck.

Reconnecting with real health doesn't mean going backwards or rejecting modern life. It means **choosing more wisely within it**. It means asking: what supports my body today? What restores balance? What keeps me steady instead of spiraling?

And importantly, it means accepting that health isn't an endpoint. It's a moving target—something you return to again and again, like a compass that helps you navigate life, not a destination you arrive at and forget.

A Simple Lens, A Big Shift

Once you begin seeing health as your body's ability to respond and adapt, the choices you make each day start to look different. It's not about achieving a perfect diet, hitting a step goal, or meditating flawlessly. It's about supporting your system so it can support you.

For some, this shift means slowing down instead of pushing harder. For others, it means reintroducing forgotten habits—like eating mindfully or sleeping without screens nearby. For all of us, it means turning out the noise long enough to hear what our own bodies are asking for.

You'll hear a lot of advice in this book. But none of it matters if it doesn't serve you. That's the core truth of real health: you are the expert of your experience. And the more you trust yourself, the more clarity you'll find.

Looking Ahead

In the next chapters, we'll explore each pillar of health—not as abstract theories, but as practices that can live inside your everyday life. The goal is not to give you more things to juggle, but to offer ways of thinking and doing that make health feel less like a battle and more like a homecoming.

Before we get there, take a breath. You've already done something powerful by deciding to return to what's essential.

You don't need to fix everything at once. Real health isn't about doing more—it's about doing what matters. And you're about to see just how simple that can be.

The Science of Simplicity

When most people hear the phrase "science of health," they imagine complex lab tests, genetic research, or cutting-edge medical devices. But some of the strongest evidence we have about health isn't hidden in high-tech settings at all—it's found in ordinary lives. It's in how people eat, move, sleep, and connect with others over decades. In the last chapter, we reframed health as something deeper than appearances or quick fixes. Now it's time to see why the simplest, most consistent habits are not only easier but also scientifically grounded. This isn't about reducing health to a handful of slogans: it's about understanding why simplicity works, and why it has always worked.

Why Lifestyle Shapes Longevity More Than We Think

When researchers study populations around the world with extraordinary health and longevity—such as those in Okinawa (Japan), Sardinia (Italy), or Nicoya (Costa Rica)—they're not looking at people who follow a single diet book or fitness plan. They're observing communities whose everyday routines align naturally with the body's needs.

These groups don't have much in common at first glance. Their cuisines, climates, and traditions differ widely. But when scientists strip away the cultural details, certain themes emerge: regular movement, mostly unprocessed foods, deep social ties, a sense of purpose, time outdoors, and consistent rest. None of these are exotic. None are expensive. But together they shape a pattern that supports long-term health.

Modern research confirms this. Large cohort studies, such as those published in *The Lancet* and *JAMA*, repeatedly show that people who engage in basic healthy behaviors—like not smoking, eating a balanced diet, moving regularly, maintaining healthy body weight, and getting enough sleep—tend to live longer and experience fewer chronic conditions. These aren't guarantees, of course. Genetics and luck play roles too. But the weight of evidence suggests that lifestyle is a powerful determinant of how well we age and how we feel along the way.

It's tempting to think longevity must come from secret protocols or cutting-edge interventions. In reality, it's often the accumulation of small, unglamorous choices that makes the biggest difference. Like compound interest, the benefits build quietly over time.

What the Evidence Really Says (and Doesn't Say)

If you've spent time online, you've seen conflicting headlines: one day coffee is harmful, the next it's protective; one day eggs are a heart risk, the next they're a superfood. These contradictions make it seem as though science itself can't be trusted. But most of the time, the issue isn't the science—it's how it's presented.

Individual studies are like puzzle pieces. Alone, they don't tell the whole story. Some are done on animals, some on small groups, some for short durations. When journalists or influencers take one study and turn it into a sweeping claim, confusion spreads.

What matters more is the **body of evidence**—what multiple high-quality studies over years consistently show. And across nutrition, exercise, sleep, and stress, the picture is remarkably steady:

- Diets rich in vegetables, fruits, legumes, whole grains, and moderate protein sources tend to support better long-term health than diets dominated by ultra-processed foods and added sugars.
- Regular physical activity—whether walking, cycling, strength training, or a mix—improves cardiovascular health, metabolic function, and mood.
- Adequate sleep supports everything from cognitive performance to immune resilience.

- Chronic, unrelieved stress can erode both physical and mental well-being, while practices that promote relaxation and connection may buffer its impact.

Notice these are broad patterns, not rigid rules. Within them, there's room for cultural diversity, personal preference, and adaptation. One person may thrive on Mediterranean-style eating; another may feel best with more rice and legumes. One may enjoy running, another dancing, another yoga. Science doesn't point to one perfect lifestyle: it shows us a set of principles we can apply flexibly.

Another thing evidence tells us is that **consistency beats intensity**. Sporadic bursts of extreme dieting or exercise rarely outperform moderate, sustainable habits. This is why so many health "transformations" revert once the program ends. The body thrives on rhythm. A little, done regularly, often has more impact than a lot, done occasionally.

A Simple Framework for Daily Living

Knowing what the evidence says is one thing. Living it out is another. The key is to translate broad principles into daily actions without feeling trapped by perfectionism or being overwhelmed by choices. Think of health like tending a garden. You don't have to understand every detail of soil chemistry to keep plants thriving. You need only a few core practices—watering, sunlight, nourishment—and a watchful eye. Over time, small consistent care yields strong roots. The same is true for your body.

Here's one way to frame it: each day, ask yourself if you've given your body the basics it needs to do its job. Did you eat food that nourishes you rather than depletes you? Did you move in a way that keeps you capable? Did you give your system time to rest and reset? Did you connect with something or someone that makes life meaningful? This isn't about scoring points or hitting targets. It's about checking in. Some days will go well, others less so. The point is to build a rhythm, not a rulebook. Over time, these check-ins become habits, and habits become part of your identity.

Take an example: imagine a person who eats lunch at their desk, rushes from task to task, and rarely moves. They may feel too busy to "be healthy." But what if they started by walking ten minutes after lunch, preparing a simple but balanced breakfast instead of skipping it, or turning off screens thirty minutes earlier at night? These aren't dramatic changes. Yet research shows even small shifts like these—especially when maintained—can support improvements in blood pressure, mood, and energy over time.

This is the science of simplicity in action: working with your biology rather than against it, aligning small daily choices with how your body actually functions.

Why Simplicity Works

Complex systems—whether ecosystems, organizations, or bodies—tend to operate best when their basic inputs are steady and supportive. The human body is no exception. It's constantly repairing, balancing, and adapting behind the scenes. When you provide stable conditions—nutrient-dense food, movement, adequate rest, manageable stress—the system can self-regulate more effectively.

This is not magic. It's physiology. For example, moderate exercise can improve insulin sensitivity, which helps regulate blood sugar. Consistent sleep can support hormonal rhythms that influence appetite and energy. Time spent outdoors may help synchronize circadian clocks and boost vitamin D. These are not one-off hacks but ongoing relationships between behavior and biology. Simplicity also reduces decision fatigue. The more rules and restrictions you impose, the harder it becomes to sustain them. By focusing on a few core principles rather than dozens of details, you free up mental energy for life itself.

Real-Life Example: Two Paths

Picture two friends, Anna and Leo. Anna follows a new diet every few months. She cuts out entire food groups, buys expensive supplements, and tracks every calorie. When she slips, she feels guilty and starts over. Leo, on the other hand, doesn't follow a named diet. He simply cooks most of his meals from whole ingredients, walks or cycles to work, goes to bed around the same time, and meets friends for dinner once a week.

Five years later, who's more likely to feel steady, energetic, and resilient? The science suggests Leo's approach, though less dramatic—may support better long-term outcomes because it's consistent, enjoyable, and sustainable. Anna's cycles of restriction and relapse may undermine the very health she's trying to build.

This isn't to shame Anna or glorify Leo. It's to show how simplicity isn't laziness; it's strategy. It's working with human nature, not against it.

Taking the Long View

One of the most liberating ideas in health science is that it's rarely too late to benefit from change. Studies of older adults show that even modest increases in activity or improvements in diet quality can reduce risk factors and improve quality of life. While early habits matter, your body remains adaptable at any age. This long view also protects against all-or-nothing thinking. If you miss a workout or eat poorly one day, it's a blip, not a failure. What shapes outcomes is the pattern over months and years, not a single moment.

By focusing on patterns, you give yourself room to experiment. Maybe you try preparing lunch differently this week. Maybe you commit to a walk at a regular time. Maybe you experiment with dimming lights earlier to help sleep. These aren't punishments, they're opportunities to learn how your body responds.

Putting Science Into Your Daily Life Without Overthinking

If the word "science" makes you think of formulas and complexity, think instead of feedback. Science at its best is a process of observation and adjustment. You can do the same with your own habits. Notice how you feel after different meals, different types of movement, different bedtime routines. Use that feedback to make small adjustments.

For instance, if you feel sluggish after heavy lunches, try lighter ones with more vegetables and proteins and see how your afternoon energy changes. If you notice your sleep improves when you avoid screens before bed, make that a small evening ritual. You're not conducting clinical trials—you're learning your own patterns. This is how you integrate evidence-based principles with personal experience.

Building on Simplicity

The science of simplicity isn't about doing less for the sake of it. It's about identifying what actually matters and doubling down on that. The evidence across cultures and decades points to the same fundamentals: balanced eating, regular movement, adequate rest, stress regulation, and social connection. Within those fundamentals, you have freedom to shape habits that fit your life, your tastes, and your circumstances.

As we move into the next chapters, we'll dive deeper into each pillar—not as rigid prescriptions, but as living practices. You'll see how nutrition, movement, sleep, and stress management can be woven into daily life without overwhelm. The goal isn't perfection; it's alignment. When your choices line up with how your body naturally thrives, health becomes less of a puzzle and more of a partnership.

Your Body, Your Baseline

Many people today live in a state of near-constant disconnection from their bodies. We've been taught to rely on numbers, apps, and outside advice to tell us how we're doing: how many calories we've eaten, how many steps we've taken, how many hours we've slept, what our macros say, or what a wearable tells us about our stress levels. Technology can be helpful—it can reveal patterns we might not notice otherwise—but overreliance on external data can dull our own internal awareness.

That inner awareness—what your body is telling you moment to moment—is often the first thing to go when life gets busy or health becomes a project rather than a relationship. But learning to tune into your body is not only possible, it's essential. Because no matter how many charts or trackers you follow, **your body already knows what it needs.**

This chapter is about reclaiming that relationship. It's about learning to recognize your baseline: the signals your body sends when things are working—and when they aren't. It's about developing a kind of trust with yourself that no expert or device can replace.

Your Body Has a Language—Are You Listening?

Think back to a time you felt truly well. Maybe you woke up clear-headed without an alarm. Maybe your digestion was quiet and unnoticeable. Maybe your energy was steady throughout the day, without needing caffeine or sugar to get through. These aren't grand moments, but they signal something important: your system was in balance.

Now think of the opposite. Days when you felt wired but tired, foggy, or short-tempered for no clear reason. Times when you had aches, bloating, headaches, or cravings that didn't make sense. These experiences are not random—they're communicating with your body. The challenge is, most of us never learned how to interpret those messages.

21

We live in a culture that encourages pushing through. Headache? Take a pill. Tired? Drink another coffee. Low mood? Scroll until it lifts. These habits may offer temporary relief, but they also train us to override early warning signs. Over time, that disconnection can make it hard to know how we really feel, let alone what to do about it.

Listening to your body doesn't mean obsessing over every sensation. It means developing an ongoing dialogue. Like any good relationship, it starts with noticing, then builds with curiosity and consistency.

Biofeedback: The Body's Built-In Dashboard

The term "biofeedback" often brings to mind specialized equipment or clinical settings, but in its simplest form, it just means noticing how your body responds to what you do. And it's happening all the time.

When you feel your heart race after a tense conversation, that's biofeedback. When your stomach churns before a big event, or your mood lifts after a walk, or your body feels stiff after hours at a screen, those are signals. They don't always need interpretation or action, but they're information. Your job is to become aware of the patterns.

Let's say you notice that after certain meals, you feel mentally sluggish or bloated. That's not guilt—it's data. You're not "bad" for eating that food. You're simply getting a message. Or maybe you find that working out late in the evening leaves you feeling restless at bedtime. That's useful to know. Biofeedback doesn't come with a flashing light or a detailed report—it arrives quietly, through shifts in energy, mood, digestion, focus, and physical sensation. Once you start paying attention, you begin to notice the subtle cues your body sends every day. Over time, these cues help you make better choices—not based on what someone else says is optimal but based on what actually works for you.

Finding Your Baseline

Everyone has a baseline—the state your body returns to when you're not under acute stress, sleep-deprived, or overloaded. For some, that baseline feels energized and focused. For others, it may involve persistent tension, fatigue, or discomfort. The baseline isn't fixed, but it reflects your current norm. Understanding your baseline helps you notice when something shifts. If you're normally clear-headed in the mornings but suddenly start waking up groggy, that's a clue. If your digestion is usually reliable but starts acting up after travel or a new work schedule, it might be worth exploring. These aren't red flags, they're signposts. They point to areas that may need more care or adjustment.

It's important not to judge your baseline. You're not trying to meet an ideal—you're learning where you are so you can navigate forward. Think of it like a compass. If you don't know your starting point, it's hard to find your direction.

Tracking your baseline doesn't require spreadsheets or wearables. It can be as simple as a few minutes of daily reflection. Did you sleep well? How was your mood? Any unusual tension, cravings, or energy dips? Over time, these reflections reveal trends. And trends are easier to work with than isolated data points.

Why Health Isn't One-Size-Fits-All

One of the biggest misunderstandings in health is the belief that there's a single correct way to eat, move, rest, or live. This mindset shows up everywhere—diets that promise universal results, routines marketed as "ideal," influencers insisting their plan is the way. But biology doesn't work that way.

Your body is shaped by genetics, history, environment, and even your mindset. A meal that leaves one person energized may leave another sluggish. Some people thrive on early mornings; others do better with later rhythms. One person may find running deeply nourishing, while another finds it stressful. These differences aren't flaws—they're part of what makes health personal. Even within the same individual, needs change. A workout routine that felt great last year might feel draining now. A diet that once worked may no longer satisfy you. The goal is not to lock in the perfect formula—it's to stay responsive.

This is why listening to your body matters more than copying a plan. When you know how to track your own experience, you can adjust early, before issues build. You can respond to signals rather than suppress them. You can honor the fact that your version of health will never look exactly like someone else's—and that's not only okay, it's necessary.

Learning to Trust Yourself Again

One of the quiet damages caused by the modern wellness industry is the erosion of self-trust. When we're constantly told we need a plan, a fix, or an expert to tell us what to do, we start to believe we can't make health decisions without someone else's authority. But the truth is, while guidance can be helpful, **you are the one living in your body every day.** That gives you access to information no one else has. Trusting yourself doesn't mean rejecting science or going it alone. It means learning to weigh outside input against your own inner feedback. It means asking, "How does this feel for me?" instead of "What's the rule I'm supposed to follow?"

This doesn't happen overnight. If you've spent years disconnected from your body—or battling it—it may take time to rebuild that trust. Start small. Notice how you feel after different kinds of meals. Pay attention to your energy levels at different times of day. Observe what helps you wind down, what disrupts your sleep, what lifts your mood. This kind of attention doesn't require perfection. It requires patience and practice.

Think of it like learning a language. At first, you may only catch a few words. But the more you listen, the more fluent you become.

Practical Awareness in Daily Life

Being aware doesn't mean becoming hyper-focused or anxious about every choice. It's more like turning the volume up on signals that are already there. Over time, you'll begin to notice more without trying so hard.

For example, if you typically eat lunch distracted—scrolling, working, or rushing—you may not notice how the food makes you feel. But if you slow down even a little, you might realize that certain meals energize you while others make you feel heavy or sleepy. That doesn't mean you need to overhaul your diet immediately. It just means you're starting to notice. And that noticing can lead to more satisfying, informed decisions.

The same goes for movement. You may find that a short walk helps reset your focus more than another cup of coffee. Or that certain types of exercise leave you feeling grounded, while others leave you overstimulated. These observations help you build a routine that supports—not drains—you. Over time, awareness becomes self-reinforcing. You begin to notice how certain choices affect not just your body but your relationships, your creativity, your ability to cope. And from there, change becomes less about discipline and more about alignment.

When Signals Are Confusing

Of course, not all feedback is clear. Sometimes your body sends mixed messages. For example, intense cravings can be the result of stress, habit, blood sugar imbalances, or emotional triggers. Fatigue might stem from poor sleep—or from doing too little physical activity. This is where compassion comes in.

Instead of rushing to fix the discomfort, pause and observe. What else is going on in your life? Have you eaten enough? Rested enough? Been under pressure? Sometimes the signal isn't about one behavior, it's about your overall state. In moments of confusion, it's okay to experiment. Try small changes and see how your body responds. And when something feels beyond your capacity to interpret or manage, that's when outside help, from a health professional, therapist, or coach. It can be incredibly valuable. Listening to your body also means knowing when to ask for support.

Awareness Before Action

In the chapters that follow, we'll explore the pillars of health—nutrition, movement, sleep, stress, and more. But before we dive into any recommendations, it's essential to root yourself in awareness. Because no habit will stick if it doesn't resonate with your experience. And no system will work if it ignores your context.

When you learn to listen to your body, you begin to build a kind of internal compass. It doesn't eliminate the need for information, but it helps you sift through noise. You begin to notice what actually feels good: not just in the moment, but in the hours and days after. You begin to see how your choices ripple out. You begin to trust yourself again. That trust is the foundation of real health. It's the quiet confidence that you're not waiting to be fixed, you're learning how to support yourself better, one choice at a time.

Food as Fuel, Not Confusion

We live in a time where food is everywhere—recipes, debates, diet plans, grocery aisles lined with choices—and yet, despite all this attention, eating has become more confusing than ever. Should you eat fewer carbs? More protein? What about intermittent fasting, clean eating, plant-based, keto, low-FODMAP, paleo? One person's "perfect diet" is another's disaster!

What's even more frustrating is that food has shifted from something simple and nourishing into something many people fear. Meals are weighed, judged, and moralized. You're "good" if you skip dessert and "bad" if you don't. This kind of thinking drains joy from eating and can make everyday choices feel like high-stakes decisions.

But if we zoom out from all the noise, we begin to see something reassuring: **your body doesn't require perfection, it thrives on consistency, quality, and simplicity.** You don't need to follow the latest trend. You just need to give your body the raw materials it understands. In this chapter, we'll clear up the confusion and return to the basics: what your body needs from food, how to spot the difference between helpful and harmful processing, and how to build meals that support you—without rules, shame, or spreadsheets.

What Your Body Actually Needs: A Gentle Look at Nutrients

Nutrition doesn't have to mean memorizing long words or counting every gram. In essence, food serves two purposes: it provides **energy** and it provides **building blocks**. Energy comes from the calories in carbohydrates, fats, and proteins. These fuels keep your brain sharp, your muscles working, and your organs functioning. Your body constantly uses energy, even when you're resting. That's why under-eating for long periods can backfire—it's like trying to run a machine with an empty tank.

The second function is repair and maintenance. That's where **vitamins, minerals, essential fats, fiber, and amino acids** come in. These don't provide calories, but they allow your body to rebuild tissues, balance hormones, regulate digestion, carry oxygen, and fight stress.

This is where food quality matters more than quantity. A snack bar and a boiled egg may both have calories, but one may leave you hungry in an hour, while the other helps you feel nourished and focused for longer. The difference isn't just in numbers—it's in how your body uses what you give it.

Think of food like raw materials in a construction site. The body can't build stable structures from poor-quality supplies. It may try to patch things up, but the result won't be as strong. Give it what it recognizes—real, whole foods—and the work becomes much more efficient.

Whole Foods vs. Processed Foods: Understanding the Real Divide

There's a lot of talk about "clean" eating or "natural" foods, but these terms are vague and often used more for marketing than science. What actually matters is **the degree to which food has been processed—** that is, how much it has been changed from its original form.

Let's take an example: oats. Whole oats you cook yourself are minimally processed. Instant oats with added sugar and flavorings are highly processed. The first contains mostly what the plant grew; the second includes additives that change how the body reacts—faster blood sugar spikes, less satiety, and more cravings later.

Processing isn't always bad. Chopping vegetables is processing. Freezing fish is processing. Even cooking is a form of processing. But the line starts to shift when processing involves stripping away nutrients and adding in artificial ingredients the body doesn't need. Highly processed foods—those packaged snacks, sweetened drinks, and fast meals with long ingredient lists—often bypass your body's natural hunger and

28

fullness signals. They're engineered to be hyper-palatable, which makes it easy to eat more while feeling less satisfied. Over time, relying on these foods can nudge your system off balance.

Whole foods, by contrast, tend to contain the fiber, water, and nutrients your body expects. They don't come with a list of instructions because your body already knows what to do with them.

This isn't about never touching processed food again. Life is flexible, and food is part of culture and convenience. But making whole foods the **default**, and processed foods the **exception**, can help your body find its rhythm again.

A Balanced Plate, Without the Overthinking

Nutrition advice often comes with complicated charts, ratios, and plans. But you don't need a nutrition degree to build a plate that supports energy, focus, and digestion. One of the most helpful and science-backed approaches is to think in **simple components**: something to fuel you, something to satisfy you, and something to support your system.

That might look like a plate with roasted vegetables, a scoop of lentils or grilled fish, and a drizzle of olive oil. Or a warm bowl of soup with potatoes, beans, and leafy greens. Or even a stir-fry with rice, tofu, and bright peppers. What matters is not hitting perfect macros or rigid portion sizes, but whether the meal leaves you feeling **satiated, steady, and energized** for the next few hours. If you feel foggy or hungry an hour later, that's useful feedback. You might need more protein. Or more fiber. Or just a slower pace of eating.

Meals don't have to be large or fancy. They just need to be **built with intention.** When you include components that support blood sugar balance—like fiber, protein, and healthy fats—you help prevent the energy rollercoaster that so many people experience daily. That crash at 3 PM? It's often tied not just to caffeine withdrawal, but to how your earlier meals were constructed.

Another key idea: **consistency matters more than variety.** You don't need to reinvent every meal. In fact, many people find that rotating a few simple, satisfying meals helps them stay nourished with less stress. If you like oatmeal with nuts and berries for breakfast, eat it regularly. If a vegetable omelet or a smoothie works for your mornings, stick with it..

Practical Examples from Real Life

Let's look at what this might look like in practice—not as a prescription, but to show how simple meals can support your health without drama.

Take Leo, a father of two who works long days and often eats lunch in his car. Instead of skipping meals or relying on fast food, he starts preparing a container of cooked quinoa, grilled chicken, and sautéed zucchini on Sunday nights. He packs it with a piece of fruit and some nuts. The meal takes ten minutes to heat and eat. He's full for hours and no longer crashes by mid-afternoon.

Then there's Julia, a college student who used to skip breakfast and rely on vending machine snacks. She now keeps a loaf of rye bread, hard-boiled eggs, and a jar of hummus in her dorm fridge. In the morning, she grabs two slices with toppings and eats them while reviewing notes. Her focus has improved, and she's no longer ravenous by lunchtime.

Neither of these people overhauled their lives. They just started building meals from real components—foods they recognize, enjoy, and can prepare without stress. That's the kind of shift that tends to stick.

Rethinking Cravings, Hunger, and Fullness

One of the most powerful things about eating whole, balanced meals is that your **internal signals start to return.** You feel when you're hungry. You recognize when you're full. Cravings become less urgent. You stop thinking about food all day because your body is actually being fed. This doesn't mean you'll never crave something sweet or salty. Cravings are part of the human experience. But instead of controlling you, they become something you can observe and respond to.

For example, if you find yourself craving sugar every night after dinner, it might be worth looking at your overall intake. Are you getting enough calories during the day? Enough protein? Are you emotionally stressed or mentally exhausted? A craving isn't a failure, it's a message. And if you do eat something indulgent, there's no need for guilt. One meal won't ruin your health just as one workout won't build it. The patterns matter more than the moments.

Food as Relationship, Not Math

Food isn't just fuel—it's comfort, memory, connection, and celebration. It's meant to be enjoyed, not feared. But the more disconnected we become from real food, the harder it gets to trust ourselves around it. Returning to simple, whole foods is a form of self-respect. It's not about rules or labels. It's about asking: *Does this support me? Does this help me feel steady and clear?* When food becomes a way of caring for yourself, rather than controlling yourself, everything changes.

In the next chapter, we'll shift from the kitchen to the body, exploring how movement works not just as a workout but as a vital form of nourishment in its own right. But for now, let this be your reminder: food doesn't have to be a battle. It can be a quiet form of support, a steady rhythm, and—most days—a deeply satisfying part of a simple, healthy life.

Eating for Real Life

It's one thing to talk about nutrition in theory. It's another to live it in the middle of a messy Tuesday, after a long day, with no groceries in the fridge and a hungry stomach staring at the empty counter. That's the real test of how "healthy eating" fits into a person's life—not on perfect days, but in the rough, rushed, or just plain normal ones.

This chapter is about those moments. About what it means to eat well when life gets loud, unpredictable, or exhausting. Because for health to be sustainable, it can't rely on discipline alone. It has to work with real life—grocery budgets, energy levels, time constraints, family preferences, and all. You don't need to count calories, memorize nutrient tables, or follow rigid rules to eat in a way that supports your body. You need a handful of strategies that are flexible, forgiving, and rooted in real foods and real choices. And you need clarity—not from perfection, but from confidence that what you're doing is good enough.

How to Eat Well Without Turning It Into a Project

Many people start with good intentions—maybe even excitement—when they try to eat better. But quickly, that excitement can morph into anxiety. Is this the "right" thing to eat? Am I getting enough protein? Should I cut carbs? What about seed oils? This kind of overthinking often comes from consuming too much conflicting information. When you're constantly exposed to health headlines, expert debates, and social media influencers each promoting their version of "truth," it's easy to become paralyzed. You want to do the best thing, but you're not even sure what that is anymore.

The solution is not to know everything. It's to **simplify your inputs and trust your process.** Eating well doesn't mean getting it perfect every day—it means having a stable rhythm of meals that keep you nourished most of the time.

This rhythm isn't rigid. Some days, you'll cook something fresh and satisfying. Other days, you'll microwave leftovers or eat a quick snack standing at the counter. The question isn't whether it's ideal. The question is: *Does this meal support my energy, digestion, and focus?* If it does, it's working—even if it didn't come from a nutrition guide or a recipe app.

The healthiest eaters aren't the ones who micromanage every bite. They're the ones who've learned how to build meals with ease, who know what helps them feel steady, and who don't spiral when things go off-plan.

Grocery Habits That Keep You Grounded

The grocery store is where most eating habits begin. It's also where many people get overwhelmed. Shelves are filled with clever packaging, health claims, and options that blur the line between "food" and "food-like products." If you don't have a system—or at least a sense of what to look for—it's easy to walk out with a cart full of stuff that doesn't support your goals. You don't need to become a food label detective. But there's value in slowing down just enough to notice what you're buying and why. Most helpful grocery habits begin before you even walk in. Starting with a rough plan—just a mental sketch of meals you might make or staples you're out of—can shift the entire experience from impulse-driven to intention-driven.

That doesn't mean you need to plan a week's worth of meals in detail. It just means knowing that you've got a few things on hand that can turn into simple, satisfying meals: a base (like rice, oats, or potatoes), a protein (eggs, beans, fish, chicken, lentils), some fresh or frozen produce, and maybe a few pantry extras like olive oil, garlic, or canned tomatoes.

When it comes to packaged foods, ignore the marketing on the front and glance instead at the ingredients. You're not looking for perfection—

you're just checking if the item is made mostly of real food, with ingredients you recognize. If you can picture what those ingredients look like outside the package, that's usually a good sign.

Keep in mind that frozen vegetables, canned beans, and pre-chopped greens aren't "less healthy" than fresh. In many cases, they can be just as nourishing and far more convenient. Convenience isn't the enemy of health—mindless choices are. If you can combine convenience with awareness, you're already ahead.

What to Cook When You're Tired, Busy, or Broke

This is where most nutrition advice falls apart—when life gets messy. Meal plans look great on paper, but they rarely survive a week filled with meetings, kid pick-ups, late nights, or empty bank accounts. The key is to shift from aspirational meals to *functional ones*—the kind you can make with low energy, limited ingredients, or little time.

First, there's nothing wrong with repeating meals. In fact, many people find that rotating a few basic meals throughout the week reduces stress, decision fatigue, and waste. A go-to dinner could be something like a veggie stir-fry with rice, an omelet with spinach and cheese, or a soup made from frozen peas, garlic, and broth. It doesn't have to be Instagram-worthy to be effective.

Second, it helps to remove the mental pressure that meals must be elaborate. Sometimes a plate of roasted potatoes, canned sardines, and sliced cucumber is exactly what your body needs. Sometimes a piece of buttered toast with a boiled egg and an apple is a fine dinner. The trick is not judging these meals as "lazy"—it's seeing them as intentional. And when funds are tight, the same principles apply. Nutrient-dense eating doesn't have to mean expensive. Beans, lentils, oats, carrots, eggs, and frozen vegetables are often among the most affordable items in the store—and some of the most versatile. A pot of lentil stew or vegetable soup can stretch across days and still provide fiber, minerals, and satisfaction.

Finally, cooking doesn't have to mean starting from scratch. Leftovers, batch cooking, and even thoughtful assembling (like tossing together pre-cooked grains, some chickpeas, and olive oil with lemon) are still forms of cooking. You're feeding yourself. That's the point.

Tuning In Instead of Tuning Out

In hectic moments, food often becomes background noise. We eat standing up, while driving, while working, or while scrolling. And in those moments, we disconnect from the experience of eating. We may not notice how much we're consuming—or whether the meal satisfies us at all.

One of the simplest but most powerful shifts in how we eat is to bring a little attention back to the process. You don't need to turn every meal into a slow, mindful ritual. But even just sitting down, putting your phone aside, and chewing more intentionally can change how you experience food. It can help you recognize fullness earlier, enjoy flavors more fully, and even digest more comfortably. This isn't about performing the "perfect mindful meal." It's about reclaiming food as something you participate in, not just something that happens to you in a rush. The more often you're present during meals, the more naturally you'll begin to trust your body's cues about hunger, cravings, and satiety.

Letting Go of Food Guilt and Perfection

One of the hardest habits to break isn't in your fridge—it's in your mind. Food guilt is so common that many people don't even realize how deeply it's shaped their eating experience. You "shouldn't have eaten that." You "messed up again." You "failed your diet." These scripts run silently in the background, turning eating into a test you're always failing.

But here's something worth remembering: food doesn't have a moral score. You are not a better or worse person based on what you ate today. Food is just input. It has effects, yes—but those effects don't define your worth. When you begin to see meals as tools rather than tests, everything softens. A sugary snack isn't a failure, it's a choice. If that choice leaves you feeling jittery, tired, or hungry an hour later, that's useful to notice. You can adjust. No shame, just learning.

This mindset shift is crucial, especially when real life throws you off track. You'll eat on the go. You'll have emotional days. You'll make choices out of convenience or comfort. That doesn't disqualify you from being a healthy person. It makes you a human one.

The most sustainable eaters are those who can zoom out. Instead of obsessing over the last meal, they look at the week, the pattern, the trend. That wide-angle view helps them stay steady without needing perfection.

Making Eating Work for Your Life, Not the Other Way Around

Food doesn't have to be your full-time job. It doesn't have to be a project or a puzzle or a source of anxiety. At its best, food supports your life, it gives you energy, clarity, steadiness, and even joy.

This support doesn't come from rigid plans or flawless execution. It comes from rhythm. From knowing what helps you feel nourished and keeping those options close. From buying ingredients you recognize. From trusting that frozen broccoli and a can of beans still count. Eating well in real life means working with what you have, your time, your energy, your budget—and making it enough. Not perfect. Just enough.

Redifining Movements and Exercises

When people think about getting healthier, the word *exercise* usually comes up fast—and often with a sense of pressure. It's easy to picture rigid routines, intimidating gym settings, or long workouts that require gear, time, or motivation you might not always have. For many, exercise becomes something to "fit in," something done to offset calories or guilt, something approached with dread rather than desire. But movement—and here we're using the broader term on purpose—isn't just about burning energy or following a plan. Movement is one of the most natural things your body is designed to do. It's how we express strength, release stress, maintain balance, and connect with the physical world. Movement is circulation, coordination, adaptability. It's health in motion.

This chapter is about reclaiming movement as a supportive, enjoyable, and deeply human part of daily life—not a punishment or a project. You don't have to train like an athlete to feel strong, mobile, and capable. You just have to move more, often, and in ways that work for your real life.

Why Movement Matters More Than You Think

While food gets a lot of attention in the health space, regular movement may be just as vital for long-term well-being. Research continues to show that people who move consistently—not necessarily intensely, but consistently—tend to experience better outcomes across a range of systems: cardiovascular, metabolic, musculoskeletal, and mental.

You've likely heard that exercise can "help" with heart health or blood sugar, and that's true. But it's more than that. Movement is an essential *input*—a signal to the body that it needs to stay adaptable, resilient, and alive. In fact, being sedentary for extended periods may signal the opposite: that the system can slow down, weaken, or start to "decommission" certain capacities. It's not about punishment or urgency.

It's about signaling life. The body doesn't need hours at the gym to get that signal. It responds to variety, regularity, and even short bursts of engagement. A short walk, a few minutes of stretching, or lifting something heavy—all of these remind the body that it still has a job to do.

Movement also does something else that's harder to measure but easy to feel: it shifts your state. A short walk after a stressful conversation can reset your nervous system. A bit of stretching before bed can ease tension. A few squats or pushups during a long workday can wake up your focus. These moments are small, but their impact is cumulative.

Redefining Exercise: From Labels to Language

One of the barriers to moving more is the way we've categorized exercise. Words like *cardio*, *strength training*, *HIIT*, *yoga*, *mobility*, *core*—they sound technical, specialized, and sometimes out of reach. But the truth is, these are just *formats* of basic human movement.

For example, cardio is just sustained movement that gets your heart rate up—like walking briskly, dancing, or biking. Strength training? That's moving against resistance—your own bodyweight, a bag of groceries, a resistance band. Mobility? That's just moving your joints through their full range of motion—reaching, squatting, twisting. Once we strip away the jargon, we see that movement isn't complicated. It's intuitive. And when you stop worrying about doing it "right," you free yourself to move in ways that actually feel good—and sustainable.

A walk is movement. Playing with your kids is movement. Gardening, swimming, carrying laundry, climbing stairs—all of it counts. You're not checking off boxes; you're keeping your system engaged. And as that engagement builds, so does your capacity.

The Spectrum of Movement: Strength, Cardio, and Mobility

Although we're avoiding formulas, it helps to understand three basic types of movement your body benefits from—just to get a feel for how to mix them into your life naturally.

First, **cardiovascular movement**, the kind that gets your heart pumping and lungs working—supports your circulatory system, brain, and mood. You don't need long runs to achieve this. A few brisk walks a day, a bike ride, a dance break in your kitchen—these send the same signal: stay vital.

Second, **strength** supports your ability to lift, carry, push, and stabilize. Strength training doesn't have to mean barbells or gym machines. It can be bodyweight exercises like squats or pushups. It can be carrying groceries up the stairs or doing a few reps with something heavy at home. The key is resistance—challenging your muscles to adapt. And the payoff is big: stronger bones, better joint support, more energy, and reduced injury risk as you age.

Third, **mobility** —often overlooked— keeps your joints moving smoothly and your posture functional. This is where stretching, dynamic warm-ups, and mindful movement styles like tai chi or yoga come in. Even reaching overhead, turning your neck gently, or rotating your hips after sitting too long helps maintain mobility.

You don't need to schedule each category into your life like a workout calendar. What you need is to stay aware of how you're moving (or not moving) and build micro-habits that give your body the range of stimuli it thrives on.

Movement in Real Life: Examples That Make It Work

Let's take a few real-life examples to see how this looks outside of theory.

Imagine Jamal, a 38-year-old who works at a desk all day and struggles with back pain. He doesn't have time—or interest—for the gym. But he starts taking 10-minute walks after meals. He adds in five bodyweight squats every time he finishes a meeting. He stretches his shoulders against the wall when he takes phone calls. After a few weeks, he notices less tension and more mental clarity.

Then there's Ana, a retired teacher who enjoys gardening but has been feeling stiff in the mornings. She starts doing gentle movements before bed—leg swings, arm circles, slow lunges. She doesn't label it "mobility training." She just starts moving her joints again. Her stiffness softens. Her confidence grows.

Or maybe you relate to Mia, a young parent who used to run but can't find time now. Instead of quitting completely, she starts playing tag with her kids in the park. She lifts them, squats with them, and carries them. It's not structured—but it's deeply physical. And it keeps her strong. These aren't "fitness programs." They're people using what they have, where they are, to keep moving.

What About Motivation?

It's easy to say, "just move more," but what about the days you don't want to? When you're tired, stressed, or just stuck in inertia?

Here's where it helps you to think about **why** you're moving—not in terms of goals or aesthetics, but in terms of experience. What do you notice *after* you move? Do you feel clearer? Looser? Lighter in mood? Often, the hardest part is starting. But if you can remind yourself of how you tend to feel afterward, not in a vague sense, but based on your own experience, you'll be more likely to take that first step.

It also helps to **lower the barrier.** You don't need 45 minutes and special clothes. If you've got 3 minutes, start there. A few stretches. A set of stairs. A walk to the mailbox. You're not committing yourself to a performance, you're just giving your body what it's asking for.

On days when motivation disappears, movement becomes even more valuable—not because you need to "stay on track," but because it helps you reconnect with your body. Even a short session can interrupt a downward spiral. It says: I'm still here. I'm still moving.

A Note on Injury, Aging, and Adaptation

Sometimes movement feels inaccessible not because of mindset, but because of pain, injury, or limitations. In those cases, the answer is not to push through blindly, it's to **adapt intelligently**. You may need to move differently, more slowly, or with help. But the principle remains: do what you can, where you are.

If you're navigating chronic pain or mobility challenges, work with a qualified professional who can guide you safely. But don't assume that movement is off the table. Often, gentle, low-impact activity can support healing more effectively than rest alone. And for those navigating the changes of aging: movement becomes even more critical—not less. Staying active can support balance, preserve strength, and reduce the risk of falls or injury. The key is to stay consistent, not intense. Your movement practice doesn't have to look like anyone else's. It just has to be yours.

Movement as a Gift, Not a Chore

When we stop thinking about exercise as a duty and start seeing movement as a form of nourishment—like food, sleep, or laughter, it changes how we relate to it. It becomes something we get to do, not something we have to force.

You don't need a perfect routine. You don't need to follow a program or train for an event. You just need to move every day, in some way, in response to what your body needs and what your life allows. As you move forward in this book, you'll see how movement interacts with other pillars—supporting sleep, mood, digestion, and even resilience to stress. But for now, all you need to remember is this: **every time you move with intention, you're building health in real time.** Even if it's just a few steps between tasks, a deep stretch in the morning, or carrying groceries with more awareness—those moments count. They always have. In the next chapter, we'll explore another underappreciated form of health-building: *rest*. Specifically, the overlooked power of sleep, and how to make it work *for* your life instead of getting pushed to the edges.

Rest, Recovery, and the Power of Sleep

When people decide to improve their health, they often focus on what to eat or how to exercise. Sleep, if it's mentioned at all, tends to be an afterthought—something that sounds important but feels negotiable. After all, most of us are used to functioning on too little of it. You get used to yawning through the day. You make peace with the brain fog. You live with low-grade irritability and chalk it up to stress or age or caffeine withdrawal.

But sleep isn't just "rest." It's not passive or optional. Sleep is one of the most *active* biological processes your body engages in. While you sleep, your brain reorganizes itself, your immune system repairs, your muscles rebuild, and your hormones reset. If food is fuel, and movement is maintenance, sleep is the *reboot*.

And unlike nutrition or fitness, which often come with layers of choice, confusion, and conflicting advice, sleep is refreshingly simple in concept. You don't need to do more—just do less, at the right time, in the right environment.

Why Sleep Isn't Just "Nice to Have"

Let's start with what we know. Sleep affects almost every system in your body. Not indirectly—*directly*.

If you don't sleep well for even a few nights, your blood sugar may swing more wildly. Your hunger hormones can shift, making you crave more calorie-dense food. Your mood becomes more reactive. Your memory slips. Your pain threshold drops. Your immune system weakens. Even your coordination becomes less precise, which is one reason why injury risk increases when you're underslept. Over time, chronic sleep debt—meaning the slow, repeated loss of deep, consistent rest—can make these

43

effects more entrenched. You may start to feel older, slower, or "off," without realizing that sleep is part of the cause.

In contrast, when you get enough quality sleep, your system starts to harmonize again. Cortisol, melatonin, insulin, and other hormonal players fall into a more natural rhythm. Mental clarity returns. Energy is steadier. Your body's ability to recover—from both workouts and stress—improves. Even your outlook on life becomes more resilient.

None of this requires perfect sleep every night. But it does show why sleep isn't optional. It's foundational.

How Sleep Regulates Hormones, Recovery, and Energy

To understand how deeply sleep supports health, it helps to know a little bit about what actually happens when you rest.

Your body moves through sleep cycles—light, deep, and REM (rapid eye movement). Each cycle plays a different role. Deep sleep is where much of your physical repair occurs—muscle growth, tissue healing, immune strengthening. REM sleep is more mental and emotional, it's where your brain processes memory, creativity, and stress. These cycles repeat every 90 minutes or so. The quality and structure of those cycles are just as important as total time in bed. That's why five hours of fragmented sleep may feel worse than seven hours of uninterrupted rest.

Now, consider how sleep interacts with hormones.

Cortisol, the stress hormone, is naturally high in the morning and low at night—*if* you've slept well. If not, cortisol can remain elevated at night, making it harder to fall asleep and creating a vicious loop. Insulin, which manages blood sugar, also becomes less efficient with poor sleep. That's why even one night of sleep loss can make you feel hungrier and less satisfied after meals. Then there's growth hormone—released primarily during deep sleep—which supports muscle repair and fat metabolism.

Testosterone and other sex hormones are also influenced by sleep quantity and quality.

This isn't about mastering hormone charts or tracking metrics obsessively. It's about realizing that sleep isn't just recovery, it's a *regulator*. It sets the stage for your entire physiological system to work as intended.

What a Sleep-Supportive Night Looks Like

The good news is that sleep isn't complicated to support. Most of us don't need fancy tools or supplements, just fewer obstacles. A night of good sleep starts before your head hits the pillow. It's shaped by the signals you send your body throughout the evening.

Light plays a major role. In nature, darkness signals the brain to release melatonin—the hormone that initiates sleep. But artificial lighting, especially from screens, can confuse that signal. Bright, blue-toned light (like from phones, TVs, and computers) can suppress melatonin and delay sleep. That's why dimming lights and stepping away from devices in the hour before bed can make such a big difference.

Temperature matters too. Your core temperature naturally drops as you fall asleep. A cooler room—often somewhere between 16–19°C (60–67°F)—can support this shift. Heavy blankets can be comforting, but make sure the room itself isn't overly warm.

Then there's the ritual aspect. When you repeat the same basic sequence before bed—washing your face, reading a few pages, stretching gently—your brain begins to associate those actions with sleep. Over time, this becomes a *cue* that sleep is coming, helping your nervous system unwind more easily. None of this has to be rigid. You don't need to follow a checklist. But developing a gentle rhythm, a signal to your system that the day is ending—can help sleep feel less like an accident and more like a return.

Real-World Examples: What Works and What Gets in the Way

Let's look at how this plays out in real life. Carla is a nurse who works long shifts and often comes home wired, even when she's exhausted. She used to scroll her phone in bed until she felt tired, but she often found herself restless and waking up groggy. Eventually, she started turning off her phone an hour before bed and listening to quiet music instead. She didn't notice a difference at first—but after a couple weeks, her sleep started to deepen. Mornings felt less like a fog.

Then there's Jim, a software developer who struggles with racing thoughts at night. He started journaling before bed—not full diary entries, just a brain-dump of everything in his mind. The act of putting thoughts on paper helped him stop looping mentally. His body felt safer to let go.

Finally, there's Andre, who travels often for work. Jet lag and hotel rooms used to throw off his sleep for days. Now he packs a small eye mask, keeps caffeine to the early afternoon, and adjusts his schedule by a few hours before flying. He still doesn't sleep perfectly on the road, but he bounces back faster.

These aren't hacks—they're habits. Personalized, low-cost, and consistent. They show that better sleep isn't about willpower. It's about removing friction and supporting your biology.

When Sleep Is Elusive: What to Try and When to Ask for Help

Of course, even with good habits, sleep doesn't always come easily. Sometimes the mind stays active. Sometimes the body feels tired but wired. Other times, sleep comes but doesn't feel restorative. These are common experiences, and they don't always require major interventions.

When sleep feels elusive, curiosity is more helpful than control. Ask yourself: What else is happening? Are you under stress? Has your routine changed? Have you been more stimulated—mentally, emotionally, physically? Instead of forcing sleep, try creating the conditions for rest. Lower stimulation. Breathe slowly. Stretch or walk lightly in dim light. And if sleep doesn't come, remind yourself that rest still matters—even if you're awake. Lying calmly in bed is not wasted time.

And if poor sleep persists—especially if you're experiencing symptoms like snoring, gasping for air at night, frequent awakenings, or severe fatigue during the day—it's worth speaking to a healthcare provider. Sleep disorders like apnea or insomnia may require professional support. There's no shame in asking for help. In fact, it may be the most health-supportive step you take.

Letting Sleep Work for You

Sleep doesn't ask for your effort. It asks for your permission. When you step out of the way—lower the lights, quiet the noise, create a little space for stillness—your body knows what to do. It has known since before you were born. You don't need perfection. You don't need eight hours every night. You need a rhythm that supports your nervous system, a space that allows your biology to reset, and a willingness to let go. Recovery isn't a luxury. It's what allows everything else—your focus, your digestion, your energy, your workouts, your mood—to function as intended. Sleep is the most foundational form of self-care, and often the most overlooked.

In the next chapter, we'll explore another form of internal regulation: your relationship with **stress**. Not just how to "manage" it, but how to understand and respond to it in ways that support both mental and physical resilience.

Stress & Mental Fitness

Stress gets a bad reputation. We often hear it talked about as something toxic, something to avoid at all costs. "I'm so stressed" has become shorthand for "I'm failing." Yet stress itself is not the problem. The real issue is **chronic, unrelieved stress**—stress without pause, without release, without recovery. Your body is wired to respond to stress. It's part of survival. When you're faced with a challenge, whether that's an exam, a traffic jam, or an argument—your nervous system activates a stress response. Hormones like adrenaline and cortisol surge through your system, increasing your heart rate, sharpening your focus, and mobilizing energy.

In short bursts, this is not harmful, it's useful. Stress sharpens you for the moment. It gets you ready for action. Athletes know this before competition, speakers before stepping on stage, parents when a child needs them in an emergency. But the design of this stress response assumes one thing: that after the challenge, there will be **resolution**. A chance to recover. A return to baseline.

The modern problem is that many of us never get back to baseline. Deadlines, notifications, bills, traffic, worries—they accumulate into a constant low hum of pressure. Instead of rising to meet stress and then resolving it, our systems remain switched on. That's when stress stops being helpful and starts becoming wear and tear.

The Silent Cost of Stress

Stress doesn't always show up as a dramatic breakdown. More often, it's subtle. A sense of always being behind. A tightness in your chest that never quite goes away. Irritability over small things. A nagging fatigue that lingers even after a full night's sleep.

The biology behind these matters. Cortisol, the main stress hormone, plays essential roles: regulating blood sugar, modulating immune function, even helping with memory. But when cortisol is elevated day after day, it can begin to disrupt rather than support. Sleep becomes harder. Digestion gets sluggish. The immune system may weaken or become overreactive. Mood can flatten or swing.

And here's the tricky part: your body doesn't distinguish between stressors. Whether you're running from a predator, juggling childcare with work, or scrolling through upsetting news, the same systems activate. Your physiology responds as if survival is at stake—even when the stress is psychological or social rather than physical.

Over time, this "always on" state leads to what some researchers call **allostatic load**—the wear and tear on the body from constant adaptation. It's not one big event, but the accumulation of many unresolved small ones. This doesn't mean stress is dangerous by default. It means that, like any signal, it needs to be respected. Ignored too long, it grows louder, often in the form of symptoms we chalk up to aging, personality, or "just life."

Awareness: The First Form of Mental Fitness

The first step in managing stress isn't to eliminate it—it's to notice it. Too often, we push past the signs until they're shouting at us. Awareness doesn't mean judgment. It means curiosity.

What does stress feel like for you?

- Do your shoulders creep up toward your ears?
- Do you grind your teeth without realizing it?
- Does your breath become shallow and fast?
- Do you reach for sugar, caffeine, or your phone the moment discomfort rises?
- Do you overwork, or do you shut down and numb out?

These aren't weaknesses, they're coping strategies. Your body and mind are doing the best they can to protect you with the tools they know. Simply recognizing these patterns is a skill. It gives you space to respond differently instead of being swept away.

Think of awareness as building a relationship with your nervous system. The more you listen, the better you can respond. And if you notice you're constantly overwhelmed, that's not proof you're broken—it's data. It means your system needs more support, rest, or boundaries.

Stress Thresholds and Personal Context

Why can one person thrive in chaos while another crumbles under smaller pressures? It's not about willpower—it's about thresholds. Genetics, upbringing, trauma history, current resources, and even sleep all influence how much stress you can handle before tipping into overload.

A soldier trained for combat, a parent juggling three kids, and a student cramming for exams all experience stress differently. What overwhelms one nervous system might energize another. This doesn't make one person weaker or stronger—it makes them *human*. Context is everything. Understanding your threshold helps you respect your limits without shame. It also helps you see that resilience isn't about "toughing it out." It's about knowing how much weight your system can carry—and building strength gradually, just like you would with muscles.

The Physiology of Calm

If stress is a natural activation of your nervous system, calm is its counterpart. The **parasympathetic nervous system**—sometimes called "rest and digest"—is what brings you back down. It slows your heart rate, deepens your breath, and allows digestion and repair to resume.

Small, intentional practices can activate this system. They don't erase stress, but they create recovery windows. Think of it as giving your body permission to reset.

- **Breathing:** Long, slow exhales stimulate the vagus nerve, a key pathway in calming. Try inhaling for four counts, exhaling for six. Even a few rounds can shift you.
- **Movement:** Gentle stretching, walking, or even shaking out your arms can discharge tension stored in muscles.
- **Mindful attention:** Noticing the present moment—the texture of your clothing, the sound of birds, the warmth of your mug— grounds you back in your body.
- **Writing:** Putting thoughts on paper externalizes them, reducing mental load and revealing patterns.

These are not grand solutions. They're signals. They tell your body: you're safe now. You can relax.

Reframing Stress

One of the most powerful tools isn't about reducing stress at all—it's about reframing it.

Studies in psychology show that when people interpret stress as harmful, they often suffer more negative effects. But when they see stress as energy mobilized for a purpose, they cope better. This doesn't mean pretending stress is enjoyable. It means recognizing that stress is your body's way of preparing you for challenge. For example, a racing heart before a presentation could be seen as "panic," or as "my body giving me energy to perform." The situation doesn't change—but the meaning does. And meaning is powerful.

Gratitude is another reframing tool. It doesn't deny difficulty. It expands your perspective. When you pause to notice what's still steady—a supportive friend, a roof over your head, a laugh you shared—you remind your brain that stress is not the whole picture. Gratitude anchors you in abundance even when life feels scarce.

Stress and the Body-Mind Connection

Stress is not just mental—it's embodied. Muscles tighten. Blood pressure shifts. Sleep cycles alter. This is why managing stress requires both cognitive tools (how you think about it) and physical tools (how you move and recover).

Think of mental fitness like physical training:

- **Consistency beats intensity.** A few deep breaths daily is more powerful than a weekend retreat once a year.
- **Recovery matters.** Just as muscles need rest, your nervous system needs downtime.
- **Capacity builds gradually.** You can't run a marathon without training. You can't face life's pressures resiliently without practicing calm.

Practical Integration

Here's what this might look like in daily life:

- Before opening emails in the morning, take 60 seconds to breathe slowly. This sets your nervous system before the flood of input.
- After work, instead of collapsing into your phone, take a five-minute walk. Let your body transition.
- If you find yourself looping on worries at night, write them down. This signals your brain it doesn't have to keep holding them.
- When conflict arises, pause before responding. Notice your body—jaw, breath, posture. Reset before reacting.

None of these require extra hours or expensive tools. They're about weaving recovery into the fabric of your day.

The Bigger Picture: Stress as Teacher

Stress, when approached with awareness, can be a teacher. It shows you where you feel unsafe, where your boundaries are thin, where your values may be in conflict. Learning from stress doesn't make it pleasant, but it makes it purposeful.

Some stress is unavoidable—life will always bring uncertainty, loss, change. But with awareness, reframing, and daily tools, stress can become less of a constant drain and more of a signal. A signpost pointing to where care, rest, or growth is needed.

Stress, Fitness, and Resilience

Mental fitness isn't about never feeling stress. It's about capacity. The capacity to rise to challenges, and the capacity to return to baseline after. The capacity to know when to push, and when to rest.

Like a muscle, resilience builds through exposure and recovery. Too little challenge and you stagnate. Too much and you break. The sweet spot is the rhythm in between.

That's the essence of mental fitness: flexibility. The ability to bend without breaking. To face life with responsiveness rather than reactivity.

Closing Reflection

This chapter is not an instruction to live stress-free—that would be impossible, and even undesirable. Stress is part of being alive. It sharpens us, motivates us, and sometimes even protects us. The problem isn't stress itself, but the lack of recovery, rhythm, and awareness that allows it to build unchecked. Chronic, unmanaged stress gradually erodes vitality, while managed, reframed, and balanced with intentional recovery, it becomes a force you can work with rather than against.

Think of stress like weather. A storm can be destructive if it never passes, but brief storms are part of what nourishes and renews the landscape. In the same way, learning to let stress rise and fall, while giving your body and mind time to reset, turns it into something less threatening and more natural. The goal isn't to fear it or deny it, but to notice it, respect its signals, and create the conditions for your system to return to steadiness.

As you move forward, remember that mental fitness, like physical fitness, builds overtime. Each breath you take to steady yourself, each moment of gratitude you practice, each pause you allow in a hectic day—these are repetitions. They may seem small, but together they strengthen your capacity to respond to life with clarity rather than collapse.

In the next chapter, we'll shift our focus outward. Beyond your inner stress response lies the external environment you inhabit—the air you breathe, the spaces you occupy, the foods and objects you surround yourself with, and the technologies that compete for your attention. Just as stress shapes you from within, your environment shapes you from without. By understanding both, you gain the full picture of what it means to live in alignment with real health: resilient on the inside, supported on the outside.

Emotions, Habits, and Inner Health

Most conversations about health begin from the outside in. We talk about food, exercise, sleep, lab results. We track numbers. We look for symptoms. But the deeper story of health often starts from within—in the patterns of thought and feeling that shape our daily behavior long before we pick up a fork or tie our shoes. Your emotions, beliefs, habits, and identity aren't just background noise. They are part of the ecosystem that determines how you treat your body, how you respond to challenges, and how sustainable any health-related change can be. This is the part of the conversation that often gets left out, yet it may be the most powerful.

This chapter is about the inner landscape of health. Not from a self-help perspective, but from a grounded, practical one. How you think affects how you act. How you feel affects how you recover. And how you talk to yourself affects whether change feels possible.

Why Your Mindset Shapes Your Health

We all carry stories about who we are and what we're capable of. These stories are often subtle. You might not say them out loud, but they're there—guiding your choices in quiet, powerful ways. *"I'm not athletic." "I always fall off the wagon." "I'm too busy to change."* These aren't just thoughts; they're internal rules. And rules tend to shape behavior.

Mindset is the lens through which you see yourself and your options. It can be fixed—rigid, self-limiting, and resistant to growth. Or it can be flexible—willing to learn, fail, adjust, and begin again. Research has shown that people with a growth mindset are more likely to persist with healthy behaviors, even when results aren't immediate. They don't define success by perfection, but by practice. Take, for example, someone who wants to start walking daily for their health. A fixed mindset might lead them to abandon the goal after missing two days: *"I knew I wouldn't stick with it."* A growth mindset reframes: *"I missed two days, but I'm still learning. I can restart now."* That small shift protects the habit. It also protects the identity of being someone who takes care of their body.

This isn't about toxic positivity. You don't need to pretend everything is fine when it isn't. But when you understand that mindset is a tool—not a trait—you gain access to something very powerful: choice. You can begin to *choose* how you frame a setback, how you talk to yourself during stress, and how you define progress. Practical Insight: If you find yourself stuck in negative self-talk, pause and ask: *Would I say this to a friend in my position?* If not, rephrase your thought as if you were offering that friend encouragement.

Identity, Self-Talk, and Daily Decisions

There's a simple but overlooked truth about behavior change: we tend to act in ways that are consistent with who we believe we are. That's why the language of identity matters so much.

Saying "I'm trying to eat healthier" creates a very different mindset than saying "I'm someone who values nourishing food." The second version doesn't just describe a behavior—it reflects a belief about self. And belief tends to guide choices, especially when motivation fades. Self-talk is part of this. The tone and content of your inner voice shapes your relationship to challenge. Are you harsh with yourself when you slip up? Do you label yourself as lazy or undisciplined when you're struggling? Or can you offer yourself the kind of support you'd give a friend—acknowledging the struggle while staying committed to your values?

You don't need to overhaul your identity to change your habits. But you do need to *align* them. If your inner voice says you're inconsistent, you'll likely act in inconsistent ways. If you start to see yourself as someone who is learning, who is willing, who is trying—your actions begin to reflect that story. Practical Insight: Try writing out a few sentences that describe your identity in the present tense, as if you're already living your values.

For example: "I move my body because it helps me feel alive." Read it back regularly, especially on hard days.

Daily decisions are rarely made in isolation. They're made in the context of how you feel about yourself that day. That's why building a healthy internal dialogue isn't a bonus feature of health, it's a foundation.

Resilience as a Practice

Many people think of resilience as a trait: something you either have or you don't. But resilience—the ability to recover from stress, adapt to change, and keep going—is more like a muscle. And like any muscle, it strengthens with use. Practicing resilience means learning how to respond, not just react. It means noticing your patterns without being controlled by them. It means bouncing back without needing to bounce perfectly.

For example, say you've been sleeping poorly and eating in a way that doesn't make you feel great. A fixed mindset might say, *"I blew it. I always do this."" A resilient mindset might say, *"That was a tough week. What small thing can I do today to shift back toward what supports me?"" Resilience isn't about constant strength. It's about capacity— having enough space in your system to respond with intention, not just impulse. Practices like mindful breathing, gentle movement, adequate rest, and honest connection all help create that space.

Practical Insight: Build a resilience ritual. Choose one small, repeatable activity that helps you reset—like walking around the block, journaling three sentences, or doing ten deep breaths. Let it be your anchor in rough moments. You don't build resilience by waiting for life to be easy. You build it by learning how to meet life as it is, and choosing how you respond. That's where your real strength lives—not in controlling outcomes, but in owning your process.

The Health Story You Tell Yourself Matters

Real health isn't just about what you do. It's about how you *relate* to what you do. It's the inner narrative that shapes whether change feels empowering or exhausting.

You won't always get it right. That's not the point. What matters is building an internal world that can hold struggle without collapse. That can greet setbacks with curiosity. That can allow progress to be slow, human, and real.

The habits that support your health begin in your mind, your beliefs, your tone, your identity. If you want sustainable change, this is where it starts. Next, we'll turn our attention to another crucial, often overlooked aspect of health: your **physical environment.** What surrounds you can either support or sabotage your well-being. Let's look at how to make it work for you.

The Social Side of Health

For decades, the conversation about health has focused on what we eat, how much we move, and how well we sleep. These are essential, but there's another dimension that often stays quietly in the background—until it starts to crumble. That dimension is connection. We tend to think of relationships as emotional extras, the "soft stuff" of life. Yet the truth is startling: human connection is as biologically essential as food, movement, and rest. It shapes our hormones, immune system, and even longevity. The body treats isolation as a threat. Belonging, it seems, is medicine.

The modern world makes this easy to forget. We can work, shop, and even socialize online without ever being in the same room as another person. We scroll through updates about hundreds of people while rarely locking eyes with anyone. We're surrounded by information but starved for connection. And as researchers continue to uncover, the health cost of that disconnection is profound.

This chapter explores why social connection matters not just emotionally but physiologically; how loneliness reshapes our biology; and what we can do—within real life's constraints—to rebuild the sense of belonging that our nervous systems crave.

The Biology of Connection

The body is not indifferent to company. When you feel understood, supported, or simply in sync with others, your physiology shifts. Heart rate slows. Stress hormones settle. The parasympathetic nervous system—the "rest and restore" branch—activates, bringing balance to the body's rhythms.

Much of this is mediated by the **vagus nerve**, a long, wandering nerve that connects the brain to nearly every major organ. It acts as a bridge between emotions and the body. When you feel safe and connected, vagal tone increases, which supports healthy digestion, steady heart rhythm, and calm focus. When you feel isolated or threatened, that tone decreases, and your system drifts toward vigilance and inflammation. Connection literally tells your body it's safe to heal.

Then there's **oxytocin**, sometimes called the "bonding hormone." It's released when we hug, laugh, trust, or share a positive social moment. Oxytocin doesn't just make us feel warm—it lowers blood pressure, reduces cortisol, and strengthens immune function. Studies show that even gentle touch or shared laughter can trigger oxytocin release, buffering the physiological effects of stress.

And beneath these immediate effects lies a deeper truth: our species evolved socially. Early humans survived not through isolation but cooperation. Safety depended on the group—on shared vigilance, shared work, and shared care. Our biology still expects that context. When it's missing, the body interprets it as danger, activating stress pathways designed for short-term emergencies but harmful when switched on chronically. In this light, friendship, family, and community are not luxuries. They are core elements of the human design. When we connect, our biology aligns with its original blueprint.

Loneliness: The Silent Stressor

Loneliness doesn't always look like solitude. You can be surrounded by people and still feel profoundly disconnected. You can live alone and feel deeply at peace. What really matters is the quality of connection, the sense of being seen, heard, and valued. But when that sense of belonging fades, the body reacts as though it's under chronic threat.

Research over the last twenty years has revealed that loneliness is as strong a risk factor for early death as smoking or obesity. People who report chronic loneliness tend to have higher blood pressure, elevated cortisol, more inflammatory markers in their bloodstream, and weaker immune responses to vaccines. Their sleep quality suffers, and their recovery from illness slows. In other words, isolation literally gets under the skin. When the brain perceives social isolation, it shifts into a self-protective state. The amygdala, which processes threat, becomes more active. Cortisol and adrenaline increase. The immune system pivots toward inflammation, preparing for potential injury. Over time, this low-grade inflammatory state contributes to the very diseases we associate with aging: heart disease, diabetes, cognitive decline. Loneliness, then, isn't just sadness, it's an internal signal of unsafety, echoing through every system in the body.

The cruel irony is that loneliness feeds on itself. When people feel disconnected, their social perception changes—they become more vigilant for rejection, more cautious in conversation, more likely to withdraw further. This self-protective loop reinforces isolation. Breaking it requires not only reaching outward but also retraining the body to trust connection again. The good news is that the biology of connection is resilient. Just as the body adapts to stress, it can re-adapt to safety. Even small, positive interactions can start reversing the physiological imprint of loneliness.

Why Digital "Connection" Isn't the Same

Social media promised to make us more connected than ever. In a technical sense, it did: we can reach thousands in seconds. But quantity has replaced quality. We share updates, not presence. We curate images, not intimacy. And while online communities can be supportive, they often lack the sensory, emotional, and nonverbal richness that the brain and body depend on.

Neuroscientists studying online interaction have found that digital engagement can trigger the same dopamine pathways as social reward—but without the balancing release of oxytocin and the calming rhythm of face-to-face communication. It becomes stimulation without soothing. The result is a paradoxical mix of hyperconnection and deep loneliness.

This doesn't mean technology is the enemy. It means it must be used intentionally. Sending a heartfelt message, having a video call, or joining a community forum that fosters real dialogue can absolutely nurture connection. What drains us is endless passive scrolling, comparison, and exposure to curated lives that distort reality. Digital connection must supplement, not replace, embodied interaction. If you've ever felt strangely empty after a long time online, that's not weakness—it's feedback. Your nervous system is reminding you that pixels can't replace presence. A hug, a shared meal, a conversation in real time, these are irreplaceable forms of regulation.

How Connection Protects Health

In 2010, a massive review of 148 studies encompassing over 300,000 participants concluded that people with strong social relationships had a 50% greater chance of survival over time compared to those with weaker connections. That's a stronger predictor than exercise habits or body weight alone. The finding has been replicated repeatedly: relationships aren't just nice to have; they're life-extending.

Part of the reason lies in **behavioral support**. People embedded in social networks are more likely to eat well, stay active, and seek help when they need it. But another part is purely **biological**. Supportive relationships modulate the body's stress response. They blunt spikes of cortisol, improve heart rate variability (a sign of healthy nervous system balance), and strengthen immune defense. Even perceived support—believing that someone would be there if needed—has measurable effects on cardiovascular health and recovery after surgery.

Connection also influences **mental resilience**. Social support buffers depression, reduces anxiety, and improves coping with trauma. It helps the brain regulate emotions more effectively, because we are wired to co-regulate—to steady each other through tone of voice, eye contact, and empathy. This is one reason therapy, community groups, and friendships all contribute to healing in different ways: they reintroduce the experience of shared regulation. Health, then, is not only an individual pursuit. It is co-created.

Rebuilding Belonging in Modern Life

If human beings are wired for connection, why is belonging so hard to maintain? Partly because our modern lifestyle fragments it. Families are dispersed. Work and screens absorb most waking hours. Many communities no longer function as true collectives; neighbors remain strangers. The pace of life leaves little time for depth. Yet even within these constraints, connection can be rebuilt—not through grand gestures, but through small, intentional acts that restore social rhythm. Start by looking at how you already interact. Do you have conversations that leave you feeling heard—or drained? Are there people who bring calm rather than comparison? Connection doesn't require constant contact; it requires authenticity. Even one or two relationships where you can be unfiltered can anchor your health.

Belonging also grows from shared purpose. Volunteering, joining a local group, or collaborating on something that matters shifts the focus outward, from isolation to contribution. Humans bond most easily through action—through doing something together, however simple. Research on "collective efficacy" in neighborhoods shows that even casual cooperation, like greeting neighbors or watching out for one another's homes, correlates with lower stress and better well-being. In other words, community health begins with micro-interactions.

Connection doesn't have to be deep every time. Even fleeting exchanges—eye contact with a cashier, a friendly nod to a jogger, small talk with a colleague—can spark the parasympathetic system. Psychologists call these **"micro-connections."** They seem trivial, but studies show that people who engage in them regularly report higher mood, reduced loneliness, and greater sense of belonging. It's not about building an enormous social circle; it's about staying open to human moments.

From Isolation to Intention

Reconnection starts internally. Before we can reach others, we often have to soften the defenses that loneliness builds. That might mean practicing vulnerability—sharing something small but real. It might mean allowing yourself to receive help without guilt. For some, it begins with addressing shame—the quiet belief that they're unworthy of closeness. Healing social disconnection isn't about forcing friendships. It's about rebuilding trust: in yourself, in others, and in the idea that connection is safe again.

One useful starting point is to notice how your body feels around different people. Does your breath slow or tighten? Do you feel energized or drained? Your nervous system is constantly reading cues of safety and threat in social interactions. By listening to those signals, you can start choosing environments that support regulation instead of stress.

When relationships feel fractured or distant, curiosity helps more than judgment. Sometimes, connection erodes not because of malice but because of distraction, unspoken resentment, or mismatched expectations. Approaching conversations with a mindset of repair: "how can we understand each other better?"—can reopen channels that seemed closed. And when certain connections remain toxic or one-sided, letting go is also part of health. Boundaries are not barriers; they are the shape of sustainable belonging.

Community as Health Practice

In many cultures, community is built into daily life—shared meals, rituals, collective work. In modern Western societies, it often has to be reconstructed. But the effort is worth it. Communities offer what no supplement or app can: **shared meaning**. They remind us that we are part of something larger, that our existence matters beyond productivity or image.

A growing body of research on "social prescribing"—a healthcare approach where doctors recommend community activities instead of, or alongside, medication—shows that participation in group programs (gardening clubs, walking groups, creative workshops) can reduce anxiety, improve mood, and even decrease doctor visits. These findings highlight something ancient: healing happens in context, not isolation.

If you're unsure where to start, look for alignment with your interests or values. Join a class, a local initiative, a book club, or a volunteer effort. Consistency is more important than intensity. Over time, repeated shared experiences transform acquaintances into support networks. And for those who feel they have no community at all, know this: belonging doesn't begin with finding the right group, it begins with small gestures of openness. Say hello more often. Ask questions. Offer genuine appreciation. Connection grows through accumulation.

Purpose, Service, and the Wider Circle

Beyond direct relationships, there's a broader form of connection that also supports health: connection to purpose. When people feel that their actions contribute to something meaningful—raising children, helping others, protecting nature, creating art—their stress responses shift. Studies on purpose and longevity show that individuals with a strong sense of meaning live longer and recover faster from illness. Purpose acts as a stabilizer—it provides psychological coherence when life becomes chaotic. It gives a reason to care for your body, because your body becomes a vehicle for contribution.

Service amplifies this effect. Helping others, even in small ways, increases dopamine, serotonin, and oxytocin—creating what some researchers call the "helper's high." It lowers blood pressure, reduces depression risk, and builds social reciprocity. The act of giving reinforces the feeling of belonging, reminding the brain that we are part of an interdependent network. In the end, belonging isn't just about receiving connection—it's about participating in it.

Healing the Culture of Disconnection

It's easy to blame technology or modern pace, but the deeper issue is cultural. We've built societies that celebrate independence over interdependence, productivity over presence. Success is often measured in personal achievement, not collective well-being. But humans are collaborative by design. When the culture forgets that, individuals suffer quietly, believing their loneliness is personal failure rather than social symptom.

Healing begins when we reclaim connection as a form of intelligence. Emotional intelligence is biological intelligence—it helps regulate the same systems that keep us alive. Workplaces that encourage collaboration and genuine appreciation report lower burnout and higher retention. Cities that design public spaces for walking, gathering, and interaction have lower stress levels. Families that share meals regularly show better mental health outcomes in both children and adults. hese are not small effects—they are the architecture of collective well-being. Changing culture starts locally. Every smile, conversation, shared effort, or moment of understanding contributes to a wider atmosphere of health. The ripple effect is real.

Connection as Daily Medicine

You don't need to overhaul your social life to feel the benefits. You can begin today, quietly. Call someone you miss. Share a meal without screens. Walk with a friend instead of texting. Ask the barista how their morning is and listen to the answer. These gestures seem small, but they send powerful signals: I see you. I value this moment. I am part of something larger than myself.

Over time, these acts retrain your nervous system toward safety and trust. They rebuild the rhythm that modern life disrupts. And as that rhythm returns, so does vitality. Connection, after all, is cyclical. The more you offer it, the more you receive. The more you receive, the more you heal. This isn't poetic—it's measurable, observable, and deeply human.

Toxins, Technology & Your Environment

When most people think of health, they picture what goes into the body: food, movement, maybe sleep. What often goes overlooked is everything around the body, the environment we live, work, and breathe in. Your surroundings matter. Not because we should live in fear of every plastic wrapper or screen, but because your environment either supports your well-being or slowly wears it down.

Toxins, artificial light, chemicals, noise, clutter, and even the way your phone interrupts your thoughts can add invisible weight to your nervous system. You may not notice these things in a single moment. But over weeks, months, and years, they can influence how you feel, function, and recover. The good news is you don't need a cabin in the woods or a full lifestyle overhaul to clean things up. You need awareness, small steps, and a mindset of progress over perfection. This chapter isn't about becoming obsessive. It's about being intentional in ways that are doable and grounded in real life.

What Really Impacts You in Daily Life

Your environment is more than your physical location. It includes what you touch, inhale, hear, and even what you scroll through. Every day, your body navigates inputs that it was not necessarily designed to handle in large quantities. From synthetic fragrances in cleaning supplies to blue light in the evening, these inputs aren't inherently toxic in small amounts. But they can create cumulative stress if exposure is constant.

Take indoor air quality. Most of us spend over 90% of our lives indoors, and indoor air can contain volatile organic compounds (VOCs) from paint, furniture, and cleaning products. Some studies suggest that long-term exposure to VOCs *may be associated* with respiratory irritation or headaches. While the science is still evolving, especially regarding low-dose exposure, minimizing unnecessary indoor pollutants is a smart, low-cost investment in health.

Then there's noise. Constant background noise—whether it's traffic, media, or open-office chatter—can subtly elevate stress hormones and interfere with focus or sleep. You may not consciously react to noise, but your nervous system does. And of course, there's light. Exposure to bright artificial light at night can disrupt circadian rhythms. Screens aren't the enemy, but if you use them late into the evening, they can confuse your brain into thinking it's still daytime. This in turn can delay melatonin release, the hormone that signals your body to wind down. None of this means you need to be paranoid. Life is full of inputs, and your body is designed to handle a fair amount of them. But when you become more aware of what those inputs are, you gain options for adjusting your exposure—or supporting your recovery.

Reducing Chemical, Plastic, and Digital Overload

The word "toxin" gets thrown around so much that it has become nearly meaningless in some health circles. But in reality, your body does interact with substances it doesn't need or want—additives in food, residues from plastics, preservatives, micro-particles in personal care products. Most of these exposures are low-grade and individually tolerated, but some research suggests that *accumulated* exposure *may contribute* to a variety of long-term issues, depending on the individual and context.

You don't need to eliminate all plastics or chemicals. What you can do is minimize unnecessary exposure where it makes sense. For example, storing hot food in glass containers instead of plastic, choosing fragrance-free personal care products, or airing out new furniture or mattresses before regular use. These simple habits don't cost much and over time may lighten the overall burden on your system. Then there's digital overload. The average person spends more than 7 hours a day in front of a screen. That alone isn't necessarily dangerous, but the *quality* of that engagement matters. Constant notifications, doomscrolling, and blue-light exposure are a triple threat to your nervous system: they can overstimulate, dysregulate sleep, and reduce your attention span.

Rather than trying to detox from all technology, the goal is digital hygiene. Can you put your phone away an hour before bed? Can you use a physical alarm clock instead of your phone? Can you carve out time in the day to be screen-free, even for ten minutes? These practices create room for your brain to reset. Practical Insight: You don't need to get it perfect. Just start with one area of reduction—like fragrance, plastic contact with food, or screen time in the evening. Let awareness guide small shifts, and trust that over time, these shifts accumulate.

Supporting the Body's Natural Detox Systems

Your body is already detoxing—right now, in fact. You have a liver, kidneys, lungs, skin, and a digestive system that are working around the clock to remove waste and maintain balance. The idea that you need extreme detox programs or harsh cleanses is not only misleading but often unnecessary.

Instead, think about how you can *support* the systems that are already doing the work. Hydration plays a big role. Water helps the kidneys filter waste and supports the liver's processing of toxins. Movement matters, too. Regular physical activity increases circulation, which helps transport waste through the lymphatic system. Nutrition supports detoxification as well. While no single food is a magic bullet, a diet rich in fiber, whole plants, and adequate protein provides your liver with the nutrients it needs to process and package toxins for elimination. Cruciferous vegetables like broccoli and kale *may help* support these pathways, but the key is overall consistency, not singular superfoods. Sleep is another overlooked component. The brain has its own waste-clearing system, called the glymphatic system, which is most active during deep sleep. That's one reason poor sleep can leave you feeling foggy—it's not just fatigue; it's your brain missing its cleanup window.

Breathing also plays a detox role. You exhale carbon dioxide and volatile compounds with every breath. Practices like deep breathing or time in nature can assist this natural rhythm, not by removing toxins per se, but by activating the parasympathetic nervous system—which helps regulate all other functions, including digestion and elimination.

Practical, Safe Ways to "Clean Up" Your Life

Cleaning up your environment doesn't need to be extreme. It's about sustainable, low-effort shifts that reduce exposure without creating anxiety. Think of it as editing your inputs rather than trying to control every variable. Start with what you notice most. If fragrance-heavy products give you a headache, try going unscented. If your sleep suffers, dim the lights after sunset or install a blue light filter on your devices. If your kitchen is full of plastic containers, replace a few at a time with glass.

It can also help to build new habits around air and water quality. Opening windows regularly (even in cold weather), adding houseplants that may support air filtration, or using a water filter (if needed in your area) are all easy steps. Again, this is not about fear. It's about lifting invisible weight off your system so that it can do its job more efficiently. And don't underestimate the impact of clutter. Physical clutter can mirror mental clutter. When your space feels chaotic, your mind often does too. Creating a calm corner—a clean desk, a tidy kitchen, a screen-free bedroom—can reduce low-grade stress and improve your sense of agency.

Digital clutter counts, too. Try turning off non-essential notifications, removing apps you don't use, or scheduling one screen-free hour a day. These small acts can create surprising relief. Practical Insight: Environmental change works best when it doesn't disrupt your life, but rather smooths it. Look for friction points, the places where your surroundings feel like they're working against you. Start there.

Shape What Shapes You

You don't live in a vacuum. The air you breathe, the light you see, the media you consume, and the objects you touch all have subtle effects on your biology and mindset. This isn't about control or perfection. It's about influence. Your environment will shape you—so you might as well shape it back. Cleaning up your life isn't about removing all risk. It's about reducing unnecessary burden so your body and mind can do what they're built to do: maintain balance, adapt, and heal.

The Real Health Reset

If you've made it this far in the book, you're not looking for gimmicks. You're not chasing a seven-day juice cleanse or a 30-day "shred plan." You're looking for something more grounded: a way to reconnect with your body when life feels noisy, scattered, or off track. That's exactly what this chapter offers: **a two-week return to the foundations of real health.** Not a punishment. Not an elimination diet. Not a rigid schedule. Instead, a chance to remove some of the static, return to basics, and rebuild momentum.

Think of it like hitting "reset" on your phone—not because the phone is broken, but because clearing away the glitches helps it run the way it's meant to. Your body is not broken. It may just be cluttered with fatigue, overstimulation, or habits that no longer serve you. This reset is a way of gently clearing the clutter.

Why 14 Days?

You may wonder: why two weeks?

The answer is partly practical. Fourteen days is long enough for you to feel real changes—better sleep, steadier energy, clearer focus—yet short enough to feel approachable. Psychologists who study habit formation note that small, repeated actions, even over just two weeks, can create new grooves in behavior. It's also a manageable timeframe for experimenting. A month-long plan can feel daunting, especially if life throws curveballs. Two weeks gives you structure without the pressure of perfection. At the end, you can extend, adapt, or simply return to your usual routine with new awareness.

The Science Behind a Reset

This reset works because it leans on the **foundational rhythms of biology**:

- **Food:** Nutrient-dense, minimally processed meals stabilize blood sugar, support gut health, and provide steady energy. Even short-term shifts toward whole foods can influence mood, digestion, and cravings.
- **Movement:** Daily activity helps regulate stress hormones, improve circulation, and sharpen cognitive function. You don't need intense workouts—consistent movement is what matters.
- **Sleep:** Quality sleep recalibrates everything: immune function, hormone balance, memory, and emotional regulation. Within days of better sleep hygiene, most people notice differences in focus and mood.
- **Mindset:** Stress management and emotional awareness calm the nervous system. Practices like journaling, mindfulness, or gratitude activate the parasympathetic system, reducing the wear and tear of chronic stress.

By weaving these pillars into your daily rhythm for 14 days, you give your body a break from the constant push-pull of modern living. It's not about restriction—it's about restoration.

The 14-Day Simple Reset Plan

Think of this reset like a **soft landing pad**. It's not about getting everything right, but about having a reliable framework to return to each day. Each day focuses on four touchpoints:

1. **Food** – nourishing without obsessing.
2. **Movement** – connecting to your body through activity.
3. **Sleep** – creating rituals that support rest.
4. **Mindset** – checking in emotionally and mentally.

Instead of rigid instructions, you'll use a **Daily Practice Template**. This creates structure while allowing flexibility.

Daily Practice Template

Each morning, ask: *What does nourishment look like for me today?*

It doesn't mean strict meal plans. It means awareness. Maybe it's packing lunch instead of relying on takeout. Maybe it's making sure your plate includes color—greens, reds, oranges from real plants. Maybe it's drinking water before coffee.

Science supports even these small changes. For example:

- Including protein at breakfast can stabilize blood sugar and reduce mid-morning cravings.

- Pairing fiber (like beans, oats, or vegetables) with meals slows digestion, promoting steady energy.

- Hydration affects cognition—studies show even mild dehydration can reduce focus and mood.

Your food choices don't have to be flawless. Aim for **real over perfect.**

Movement: Consistency Over Intensity - Daily movement isn't about grinding at the gym. It's about keeping your body in rhythm. This could be a brisk walk, bodyweight stretches, dancing in your living room, or yoga before bed.

Research shows that just 20–30 minutes of moderate activity daily can improve sleep, reduce stress hormones, and support cardiovascular health. The form doesn't matter as much as the rhythm.

Ask yourself: *What kind of movement would help me feel more alive today?*

Sleep Rituals: Preparing to Power Down - Sleep is not just "rest." It's an active state of repair. During deep sleep, your brain clears waste products, your immune system recalibrates, and your muscles rebuild.

To support this, create a **wind-down ritual**: dimming lights, turning off devices, sipping herbal tea, or reading. Even 10 minutes of intentional routine tells your nervous system it's safe to shift gears.

Tip: Research shows that exposure to blue light in the evening delays melatonin release, making sleep harder. If you can, reduce screen time 30–60 minutes before bed.

Mindset & Self-Check: Listening Inward - Stress often lingers because we don't pause to notice it. A daily check-in grounds you. Ask:

- *What am I feeling physically?*

- *What emotions am I carrying?*

- *What do I need most right now?*

This isn't a test—it's a conversation with yourself. Over time, this builds **interoception**—the ability to sense what your body is experiencing. Studies suggest that people with higher interoceptive awareness often regulate emotions better and make healthier choices.

What to Expect (And How to Adjust)

The first few days may feel bumpy. If you're used to late nights, sugar, or constant screen time, your body might resist. You may feel tired as your sleep rhythm resets. You may notice cravings when you eat fewer processed foods. This isn't failure—it's adaptation. Your body is recalibrating. Think of it like shifting from running on fumes to running on steady fuel.

By the end of the first week, many people notice:

- Clearer mornings, less grogginess.
- More stable energy (fewer afternoon crashes).
- Improved digestion.
- A sense of calm from daily check-ins.

But remember—everyone adapts differently. If a day falls apart, don't throw away the plan. Ask: *What's one small thing I can do today to feel more aligned?* Then do that.

Practical Tips for Success

- **Start simple.** Don't overhaul everything at once. Choose one pillar to emphasize the first few days.
- **Use cues.** Link new habits to existing ones. For example, stretch after brushing your teeth, or write your self-check while the coffee brews.
- **Make it enjoyable.** If movement feels like punishment, you won't sustain it. Choose activities that bring pleasure.
- **Forgive lapses.** Consistency, not perfection, drives change. A missed day doesn't erase progress.

The Power of Returning

By the end of 14 days, your life may not look dramatically different. But you may notice something subtle but profound: you feel more attuned. You're clearer on which foods steady you, which movements energize you, which rituals help you rest. This reset isn't meant to be a one-time challenge. It's meant to be a **framework you can return to anytime.** After travel, illness, or stressful seasons, you can use this same rhythm to find your footing again. Real health is not a destination. It's a practice of returning—again and again—to what supports you.

In the next chapter, we'll explore how to carry these rhythms forward, not just for two weeks, but for the long arc of your life. Because the real gift of this reset isn't just feeling better now—it's remembering that you always have the power to begin again.

Life After the Reset

Two weeks of intentional practice can shift your energy, clear some mental fog, and remind you of how good your body and mind are capable of feeling. But real health is built in the weeks, months, and years that follow. Not because you're always "on" or hyper-disciplined, but because you learn how to stay steady when life throws you off.

This chapter is about the part most health books skip: what happens *after* the plan. When the structure fades, motivation dips, and real life—with its stress, travel, emotions, and curveballs—comes rushing back in. This isn't where your progress ends. It's where it becomes real. True health is not the reset. It's your ability to return to what matters, again and again, with less drama and more ease.

Making Healthy Your New Normal

A sustainable health routine isn't about heroic effort. It's about design. It grows from small, repeatable choices that feel like a *fit* for your actual life. After the reset, your job isn't to maintain some perfect version of the plan. It's to ask: *What parts of this feel natural enough to keep going?*

For some, it might be the morning walk. For others, it's cooking at home more often, or turning off screens an hour before bed. What sticks tends to be what feels *supportive*, not what feels *forced*.

Try not to measure success by how closely you follow a plan. Measure it by how well your routines support your energy, clarity, and capacity to handle daily life. If a habit helps you show up with more steadiness, it belongs. This is the difference between a "health kick" and a lifestyle. You're not chasing outcomes anymore. You're building a foundation— and foundations are supposed to feel solid, not exhausting.

Practical Insight: Ask yourself once a week, *What health habits felt most helpful this week?* Then reinforce those, instead of fixating on what you missed.

Navigating Change Without Guilt

Life doesn't stay the same for long. Jobs change. Routines shift. Motivation fades. The old model of health—where you find the "perfect plan" and stick to it no matter what—just isn't built for real life. Instead, think of health as a relationship. Sometimes you're close and consistent. Other times, you drift. But just like in any relationship, what matters is the ability to reconnect without shame. Guilt can be a toxic part of health culture. Miss a workout? Eat a takeout meal? Sleep poorly? The goal isn't to punish yourself. It's to notice how it felt, reflect, and recalibrate. You don't need to start over. You just start *again*.

A useful question in any health setback is: *What would support me right now?* Sometimes that support looks like a nourishing meal. Sometimes it's a long nap. Sometimes it's just letting yourself off the hook. Your needs aren't static, and neither should your habits be. Practical Insight: When you catch yourself feeling guilty for falling off track, pause. Say aloud: *This moment is an invitation to begin again.* Then do the next helpful thing—nothing more, nothing less.

Tracking Progress Without Obsession

The desire to "measure" progress is natural. We want evidence that our efforts are working. But health is more than numbers. It's how you feel when you wake up. How clearly you can think. How quickly you bounce back from stress. And yes, sometimes those changes are too quiet for data to capture. That doesn't mean tracking is bad. It just means the *intention* behind it matters. If you enjoy journaling your workouts or meals, do it. If you wear a fitness tracker that motivates you, great. But be careful not to hand over all your authority to a device or a data sheet. Your body's signals matter just as much—often more.

Tracking becomes harmful when it fuels anxiety, shame, or comparison. It becomes helpful when it gives you feedback, not judgment. So how can you stay connected to your progress without obsession?

- Reflect weekly on your energy, mood, and sleep.
- Notice how you feel *in your body*, not just how it looks.
- Celebrate consistency over intensity.

Practical Insight: At the end of each week, write down one health-related moment you felt proud of. It could be a decision, a feeling, a shift in mindset. This builds positive reinforcement without pressure.

Carrying Simplicity Forward

The end of the reset isn't a finish line. It's an invitation. To live in a way that feels more aligned. To be gentler with yourself. To stay curious, even when progress feels slow. Real health doesn't come from knowing more. It comes from doing less—with more intention. Returning to the basics. Noticing what works. Letting go of what doesn't. And remembering, always, that your body is on your side. In the next chapter, we'll explore common roadblocks, real-life scenarios, and how to troubleshoot without shame. Because even the most thoughtful routines need adjusting sometimes. And that's not failure. That's life.

When Things Get Hard

If you've ever tried to create healthier habits and found yourself thrown off course by a long day, a cold, or a stressful week—you're not doing it wrong. You're doing it exactly the way real life unfolds. Health isn't measured by how well we do when things are easy. It's shaped by how we respond when things get hard. This chapter is about what happens when momentum fades, plans unravel, and you find yourself in the very human space between intention and reality. Setbacks are part of the process, not the end of it. Let's explore how to meet them with more curiosity than criticism—and how to rebuild with less pressure and more grace.

What to Do When You Slip

At some point, you will skip the walk, grab the drive-thru meal, stay up too late scrolling, or just lose your rhythm completely. It happens. The goal isn't to avoid slipping, it's to make your recovery easier, faster, and less emotionally loaded.

The first step is to notice the moment without judgment. Slipping doesn't mean starting over. It doesn't undo the progress you've made. One off day—or even a string of them—is not a failure. It's just a pause. You haven't lost everything. You're just momentarily disconnected from your routine. Often, the instinct after a slip is to either give up completely or swing to the other extreme: doubling down with stricter rules, detoxes, or punishment workouts. Neither approach is helpful. What you need is a soft return. Ask yourself: *What's the gentlest, most helpful next step I can take today?* It might be a glass of water. A short walk. A meal that steadies your energy. One act of reconnection can reset your direction.

Stress, Sickness, Schedules, and Setbacks

Let's be honest: life is not built around your ideal health routine. It's full of surprises. The question isn't if stress, illness, or time crunches will show up, it's how you respond when they do.

Stress can derail habits quickly, especially if health practices were built during calmer times. You may find yourself stress-eating, skipping movement, or losing sleep. Rather than trying to maintain your full routine, focus on micro-habits. If your nervous system is on edge, a five-minute walk or five deep breaths may do more good than forcing yourself through a workout. Health under stress is about regulation, not intensity.

Sickness changes the picture entirely. When you're not well, your body needs rest, fluids, and patience—not discipline. Forcing yourself to move or eat "perfectly" through illness often slows recovery. The best support you can offer your body during sickness is permission to heal. When energy returns, so can structure.

Schedules don't always respect your best intentions. Maybe a project swallows your week. Maybe your kids get sick. Maybe travel or caregiving responsibilities pull you out of routine. This is where flexible systems matter more than perfect plans. Even in a chaotic schedule, you can anchor yourself with one small health-supporting act a day: drinking enough water, packing one nourishing snack, taking a phone call while walking.

Setbacks can be emotional, not just logistical. You might go through loss, heartbreak, burnout. These moments test your resilience. Not because you should "push through," but because they ask you to listen more closely. During emotional setbacks, gentle self-care becomes essential. The practices that keep you grounded—sleep, food, breathing, movement—don't fix the problem, but they help you meet it with more strength.

Practical Insight: When life gets complicated, shift from optimization to maintenance. Don't ask, *What's the healthiest thing I could do?* Ask, *What's the kindest thing I could do that still supports me?*

How to Rebuild Quickly and Kindly

Rebuilding your rhythm after a setback isn't about willpower. It's about reducing friction.

Start small. Don't try to return to your full routine on day one. Choose one area that feels easiest to reclaim. Maybe it's making your bed. Maybe it's preparing breakfast. Choose something that signals, *I'm back.*

Then stack gently. Add one piece at a time—movement, then sleep hygiene, then meal prep. Let momentum do the heavy lifting. When you rebuild gradually, each win reinforces the next. More importantly, you avoid the all-or-nothing trap that often leads to burnout. Use visual cues to remind yourself that you're supported. Keep a journal or note on your fridge with a few phrases that ground you: *Progress, not perfection. This is what returning looks like. My health is flexible.* And be honest about what contributed to the slip. Without shame, reflect on what made your habits harder to maintain. Was it stress? Exhaustion? Lack of preparation? Emotional overwhelm? Understanding the root helps you prevent it from becoming a pattern. Some people find it helpful to build a "recovery ritual"—a short sequence that helps you re-anchor after any disruption. That might include tidying your space, cooking a simple meal, and getting to bed early. This becomes your reentry ramp, a reliable pathway back to feeling like yourself. Practical Insight: Design your own "reset day" script. Not a punishment, but a calming rhythm you can return to when life feels frayed.

Resilience in Real Time

Health isn't about never falling down. It's about rising without panic. Responding instead of reacting. Choosing again, even when it would be easier to numb out. When things get hard, let that be your cue to come closer to yourself—not farther. Let your health habits flex with life, not fight it.

Setbacks are not shameful. They're built into the architecture of real life. And every time you meet one with patience, self-respect, and a gentle return, you strengthen the core of what health really is: not performance, but resilience.

In the next chapter, we'll shift from personal setbacks to common questions—addressing the real-world challenges that so often trip people up. Because knowing how to troubleshoot is just as important as knowing how to start.

Troubleshooting & FAQs

Most people don't fall off track because they lack desire. They fall off because something gets in the way. A logistical snag, an emotional trigger, an unexpected roadblock. You know what to do, but life interrupts. This chapter is about navigating those interruptions—not with discipline, but with understanding. The questions in this chapter are the ones people ask quietly when they feel like they're the only one struggling. You're not. These are normal challenges, and working through them is part of building a sustainable approach to health. Let's address the big one.

What if I Don't Have Time?

Time is one of the most common reasons people abandon healthy routines. The truth? You probably *don't* have time to do everything. But that doesn't mean you can't do something. The key shift is to stop seeing health as an "add-on" and start seeing it as part of the infrastructure that supports your day. You don't need an hour for the gym or a meal prep Sunday to stay on track. You need a few reliable anchors.

If mornings are hectic, maybe breakfast becomes a smoothie you blend while your coffee brews. If evenings are packed, maybe movement comes in the form of walking during phone calls. These are actual strategies. Instead of aiming for "ideal," look for "available." And remember, even five minutes of focused attention can shift your mood, energy, and mindset. That matters. Practical Insight: When time is tight, anchor your day with a single habit you can do without overthinking. One glass of water. One stretch. One minute of quiet.

What If I Struggle With Cravings?

Cravings are not character flaws. They're signals—sometimes from your body, sometimes from your emotions. Ignoring them doesn't always work. But learning to listen differently does.

Biologically, cravings may reflect nutrient imbalances, blood sugar dips, or inconsistent meals. Emotionally, they often show up in response to stress, boredom, loneliness, or habit loops. The next time you experience a strong craving, pause. Ask: *What am I actually needing?* Sometimes you do need the chocolate. Sometimes you need rest, or a walk, or someone to talk to. When you meet the real need, the craving often softens. And if you choose to eat the thing? Do so with awareness, not guilt. Guilt tends to prolong the cycle.

Over time, balanced meals, steady hydration, better sleep, and emotional regulation can reduce the intensity of cravings. But you don't need to eliminate them to be healthy. You need to relate to them with curiosity instead of shame. Practical Insight: Before responding to a craving, drink a full glass of water and take ten slow breaths. This creates a small space between urge and action.

What If I Can't Sleep Well?

Sleep struggles are deeply frustrating. You know you need rest, but your body or mind won't cooperate. First, know that you're not alone. Sleep issues are common and multifaceted. Sometimes the issue is *falling* asleep. Other times it's staying asleep or waking up exhausted. There is no single fix, but there are patterns that can support better sleep over time. Start by looking at the rhythm of your day. Are you spending most of it under artificial light? Are you on screens late into the night? Are you eating or exercising too close to bedtime? These can all disrupt your natural sleep-wake cycle.

Stress and overthinking are also common sleep disruptors. If your mind is racing, try a simple journaling practice before bed: write down everything that's swirling around, without editing. Get it onto paper so it doesn't stay in your head. And if you wake up during the night? Don't panic. Try progressive muscle relaxation, a breathing exercise, or reading something calming. Avoid the urge to check your phone. Your body may just need time to down-regulate.

If sleep issues persist, it may be time to consult a qualified healthcare provider or sleep specialist. There could be underlying causes worth exploring. Practical Insight: Choose one small evening ritual (like dimming lights or putting your phone away 30 minutes earlier) and repeat it nightly to signal your body it's time to slow down.

Other Common Obstacles

"I keep starting and stopping." This is not failure. It's practice. Most sustainable habits come from repeating imperfect efforts, not following perfect plans. Every time you restart, you get a little better at it.

"I don't feel motivated." Motivation is overrated. What you need is momentum. Start small. Let the feeling of doing something good create its own drive.

"My environment doesn't support me." Maybe your workplace is stocked with snacks, or your family doesn't share your goals. You don't need everyone around you to change—you just need a few cues that help *you* stay anchored. A water bottle on your desk. A prepped lunch. A walk at lunch break. Make it visible and easy.

"I feel overwhelmed by information." You don't need more data. You need a filter. Come back to the pillars you know support you: real food, daily movement, quality rest, stress awareness. If a piece of advice doesn't reinforce one of those, it may not belong right now.

"I feel discouraged." That's normal. Especially when change feels slow. But don't mistake slow for stuck. Your body responds over time, not overnight. Stay connected to your *why*, and let consistency do the rest.

The Questions Are Part of the Path

If you have questions, it means you care. You're paying attention. You want to do this well. That's not weakness. That's the start of wisdom. Troubleshooting is not a sign that something is broken. It's a natural part of growth. Real health isn't built on perfect routines. It's built on the ability to keep showing up, to keep learning, and to keep adjusting with care.

In the next chapter, we'll hear from real people who have done just that—everyday stories of simplicity in action. Because sometimes, what we need most isn't more advice. It's a glimpse of what's possible when we take it one small step at a time.

Real Stories, Real Simplicity

We often absorb information through facts and principles, but we internalize it through stories. A chart might show the benefits of sleep or walking, but a real person describing how better rest changed how they show up for their kids—that sticks. It reminds us that health isn't just about metrics or routines. It's about how we feel in our lives. This chapter isn't about before-and-after photos or dramatic transformations. It's about real people, in real circumstances, making realistic changes that supported their wellbeing in meaningful ways. Their stories aren't perfect, and that's what makes them useful. They're honest. They're grounded in everyday life. And they show what it looks like to apply the principles of this book in your own way, at your own pace.

Each story has been anonymized and paraphrased with permission to protect privacy, while keeping the spirit and details true to the person's experience.

Mateo – Finding Simplicity During a Job Change

Mateo, 38, works in tech and lives in a busy urban environment. After a major career shift that left him working longer hours and under more pressure, his energy plummeted. Meals became rushed, sleep erratic, and exercise non-existent.

"I didn't feel unhealthy," he said, "but I also didn't feel present. I was foggy all the time."

When Mateo read about the concept of "anchors" in this book—small, reliable practices that bring stability—he decided to start with one. Each morning, before checking his phone, he drank a full glass of water and stepped outside for a five-minute walk. "It was tiny, but it gave me momentum," he shared. That led to packing lunches more often, and eventually, shutting screens off earlier. He never started a workout program, never counted calories. But after a few months, he said, "I felt like I had a say in my day again." His takeaway? "Don't underestimate what five minutes can do when you repeat it."

Angela – Resetting Sleep After Years of Burnout

Angela, 44, is a night-shift nurse. Years of working odd hours left her wired at night and sluggish during the day. She assumed this was just part of the job.

"I figured broken sleep was my reality forever," she said. But after reading about circadian rhythms and gentle evening rituals, she decided to try a few changes—dimming lights post-shift, no screens in bed, and breathing exercises before sleep. The results weren't immediate. But over six weeks, her average sleep window improved by almost two hours. She still worked nights but began feeling more rested.

"I didn't realize how much my nervous system was stuck in overdrive," she shared. "Once I learned how to downshift, everything felt less chaotic." Angela's story isn't about curing sleep issues. It's about respecting them. Her small shifts supported the body she had, in the life she lived.

Jason & Lina – Redefining Movement as a Family

Jason and Lina, a couple in their early 30s with two young kids, felt frustrated with how inactive they'd become since becoming parents.

"Gyms were out of the question, and trying to coordinate workouts felt impossible," Jason said. "We kept thinking movement meant exercise." Instead of formal workouts, they started walking together after dinner with the kids. Sometimes just around the block, sometimes longer. They added short dance breaks during weekend cleanups and began stretching together before bed.

"We stopped thinking in terms of exercise and started thinking in terms of movement," Lina said. "The kids noticed too. Our four-year-old now reminds us to 'shake out our legs' if we're grumpy." What shifted for them wasn't just physical activity. It was family rhythm. Movement became part of connection, not a chore.

Sarah – Letting Go of Perfection

Sarah, 29, spent years chasing health through extremes—cleanses, tracking apps, rigid routines. "I thought if I could just follow the plan perfectly, I'd feel in control," she said. But the harder she pushed, the more stressed she became. She began experiencing sleep disruption, mood swings, and anxiety around food choices. After reading Chapter 9 on emotions and inner health, something clicked.

"I realized I was using health as a way to earn my worth," she shared.

Instead of overhauling her habits again, she stepped back. She stopped tracking. She focused on feeling satisfied after meals, moving when she needed clarity, and doing daily check-ins without judgment.

"I still care about my health," Sarah said. "But now I define it by how kind I can be to myself, not how strict." Her health improved—not by doing more, but by doing less with more intention.

Why These Stories Matter

What these stories have in common isn't perfection or discipline. It's presence. Each person started small. Each one respected their season of life. And each discovered that the path to real health isn't paved by willpower, but by self-awareness. Your story will look different. And that's the point. Real health is simple not because it's easy, but because it doesn't require you to become someone else.

Nature's Pharmacy: Foods That Support Your Body

Food doesn't just give us energy. It shapes our biology in real time. Every bite you eat sends information to your cells: messages about inflammation, immune response, hormone production, and brain chemistry. It's not just about calories in and out. It's about how the compounds in food interact with your body's systems. What makes this topic complex is that food isn't a single nutrient or ingredient. A blueberry isn't just sugar and fiber; it's also packed with anthocyanins, vitamin C, and other phytochemicals that may reduce oxidative stress. A handful of walnuts isn't just fat; it's a rich source of plant-based omega-3s, polyphenols, and magnesium.

In this chapter, we'll explore a wide range of foods—not from a moral lens ("good" or "bad") but from a functional one. What can these foods do *for* you? What does science suggest about how they might support your energy, immunity, focus, and long-term health? Importantly, this isn't about perfection or prescriptions. It's about awareness. The more you understand what's on your plate, the more empowered you are to make choices that work for *you*.

Micronutrient-Dense Foods and Their Roles

Some foods are nutrient "powerhouses" because they deliver a high concentration of essential vitamins and minerals per calorie. These nutrients often serve as cofactors for enzymes that keep your body running smoothly.

Leafy greens like spinach, kale, and arugula provide folate, vitamin K, magnesium, and plant-based calcium. Folate, for example, plays a crucial role in DNA repair and red blood cell formation.

Egg yolks are rich in choline, which supports brain health and cellular membrane function. Choline also plays a role in neurotransmitter synthesis (especially acetylcholine, which is involved in learning and memory).

Shellfish, such as oysters and mussels, are incredibly dense in zinc, vitamin B12, and selenium—nutrients that support immune health and thyroid function.

Liver (especially from pasture-raised animals) is perhaps the most nutrient-dense food gram-for-gram, offering high levels of iron, vitamin A (in its active form), B vitamins, and copper. While not everyone enjoys liver, small amounts may offer substantial nutritional benefit.

Anti-Inflammatory Foods: What Science Says

Inflammation isn't inherently bad. It's part of the immune system's response to stress or injury. But when inflammation becomes chronic and low-grade, it's linked to nearly every major chronic disease.

Many foods contain compounds that may help modulate inflammation:

- **Berries** (blueberries, raspberries, blackberries) are rich in flavonoids, especially anthocyanins, which some studies suggest may reduce markers of inflammation and oxidative damage.
- **Fatty fish** like salmon, sardines, and mackerel are high in EPA and DHA, long-chain omega-3 fatty acids that play anti-inflammatory roles in the body.
- **Turmeric**, when consumed with black pepper (which boosts absorption of its active compound, curcumin), has been studied for its potential to down-regulate pro-inflammatory cytokines.
- **Extra virgin olive oil** contains oleocanthal, a compound with anti-inflammatory properties similar in mechanism to ibuprofen (in vitro studies). It's a staple of the Mediterranean diet, which is associated with reduced risk of inflammatory conditions.
- **Green tea** offers epigallocatechin gallate (EGCG), a catechin that may support immune regulation and reduce oxidative stress.

These foods don't "fight inflammation" in a vacuum. They support your body's regulatory systems, helping maintain balance when consumed consistently as part of an overall diet.

Gut-Supportive Foods

Your gut is not just a digestive tube—it's a major immune organ, a hormone-producing site, and a key interface between food and your body's systems. A healthy gut microbiome is associated with everything from reduced inflammation to improved mental health.

Foods that may support your gut health include:

- **Fermented foods** like yogurt, kefir, kimchi, sauerkraut, and miso. These contain live bacteria (probiotics) that can temporarily boost microbial diversity.
- **Prebiotic fibers** found in garlic, onions, leeks, bananas (especially underripe), asparagus, and oats. These feed beneficial gut bacteria and help produce short-chain fatty acids like butyrate, which may support gut barrier integrity and reduce inflammation.
- **Bone broth**, rich in collagen, glycine, and glutamine, may support gut lining repair, though more human studies are needed. It also provides minerals like calcium and magnesium in bioavailable forms.
- **Polyphenol-rich foods** (berries, olive oil, green tea, cocoa) have been shown to influence gut microbial balance, encouraging growth of beneficial strains.

Brain-Boosting Foods

Cognitive health isn't just about memory or focus, it's also about emotional regulation, sleep quality, and mental clarity. Nutrition can play a quiet but significant role here.

- **Oily fish** (again, for DHA): DHA is a structural fat in the brain and retina. Some evidence links higher DHA intake to reduced cognitive decline.
- **Pumpkin seeds** are rich in magnesium, iron, zinc, and copper— minerals that support brain signaling and oxygen transport.
- **Dark chocolate** (at least 70% cacao) is a source of flavonoids that may improve blood flow to the brain and support cognitive function, especially in older adults.
- **Berries and cherries** contain compounds that may cross the blood-brain barrier and influence neuronal signaling.
- **Coffee**, in moderation, has been linked in some studies to better focus, reaction time, and reduced risk of neurodegenerative diseases. The benefits likely come from both caffeine and polyphenols.

Immune-Supportive Foods

Your immune system relies on adequate nutrient status and low inflammatory burden to work properly. No food can prevent illness, but a well-nourished body may respond more effectively to pathogens.

- **Citrus fruits** (and bell peppers) are high in vitamin C, which supports white blood cell production and antioxidant recycling.
- **Zinc-rich foods** like pumpkin seeds, oysters, and lentils play a role in immune cell signaling.
- **Mushrooms** (especially shiitake, maitake, and reishi) contain beta-glucans that may modulate immune activity.
- **Cruciferous vegetables** like broccoli, cauliflower, and Brussels sprouts contain sulforaphane, which may activate pathways involved in cellular defense and detoxification.
- **Garlic**, especially raw, has been studied for its potential antimicrobial and immune-modulating properties, though results are mixed and depend on preparation.

A Gentle Word on Superfoods

You might be wondering, what about superfoods? Kale, acai, goji berries, chia seeds? These are all nutrient-dense, but the term "superfood" is mostly a marketing tool. What matters more than any one food is *the pattern over time.*

A daily apple can be as powerful as an exotic berry if it's consistent. You don't need to chase trends. You need to build a base of real, minimally processed foods that support your body's actual needs.

Building Your Plate with Purpose

By now, we've explored how individual foods may support various body systems, from the gut to the brain. But in real life, we don't eat nutrients in isolation. We eat meals—often in social, emotional, and time-sensitive contexts. That means how you combine, balance, and relate to foods over time matters just as much as what you eat.

This chapter focuses on the big picture: how to build a plate with intention, how to think about macros without obsessing, and how to enjoy flexibility while still nourishing your body well. We'll look at protein, fats, and carbohydrates in context, touch on popular topics like sugar, caffeine, and alcohol, and help you connect food choices with your personal goals, energy, and moodIt's about rhythm.

Protein: The Most Satisfying Macronutrient

Protein isn't just for athletes or bodybuilders. It's a structural component of your muscles, bones, enzymes, neurotransmitters, and immune cells. Getting enough protein may help support satiety, muscle maintenance (especially as you age), blood sugar regulation, and recovery from stress.

Sources can vary widely:

- **Animal proteins** like eggs, chicken, turkey, fish, yogurt, and beef provide all essential amino acids and are highly bioavailable.
- **Plant proteins** such as lentils, tofu, tempeh, chickpeas, quinoa, and black beans can be excellent options, though they may require greater volume or variety to meet full amino acid needs.

The key with protein is consistency. Including a protein source in each main meal can help you stay satisfied, preserve muscle mass, and support your metabolism.

Carbohydrates: Energy and Fiber

Carbs are not the enemy. They're the body's preferred energy source, especially for the brain and during physical activity. What matters most is the *type* of carbohydrate and the *context* in which you eat it.

- **Whole food carbs** like oats, brown rice, root vegetables, legumes, fruit, and quinoa provide fiber, vitamins, and a slower glycemic impact.
- **Refined carbs** like white bread, pastries, sweetened cereals, and sugary drinks may spike blood sugar more rapidly and lack key nutrients.

That doesn't mean refined carbs are always off limits. But relying on them heavily can lead to energy crashes, hunger spikes, and poor satiety. Instead, prioritize complex carbohydrates that include fiber and nutrients, and pair them with protein or fat to slow digestion and improve energy stability.

Fiber is especially worth noting: it feeds your gut bacteria, supports regularity, and may help with cholesterol regulation. Many people fall far short of the daily recommended intake. Including fibrous foods like lentils, flaxseeds, and veggies can help bridge that gap naturally.

Fats – Hormones, Brain, and Long-Term Fuel

Fat got a bad reputation in past decades, but science has shifted. Fats are essential for hormone production, brain health, cell membrane integrity, and long-term satiety.

- **Unsaturated fats** (from olive oil, avocado, fatty fish, nuts, and seeds) are associated with cardiovascular and cognitive benefits.
- **Saturated fats** (from dairy, meat, coconut) are more debated. While moderation appears safe for most people, excess intake from ultra-processed foods may contribute to inflammation or lipid issues.

- **Trans fats**, often found in hydrogenated oils, are best minimized as they're consistently linked to inflammation and cardiovascular risks.

Healthy fats can enhance the absorption of fat-soluble vitamins (A, D, E, K) and make meals more satisfying. Including moderate fat in every meal supports mood, blood sugar, and brain clarity.

How to Think About Sugar, Caffeine, and Alcohol

Sugar isn't poison, but excessive intake, especially from sugary drinks and packaged foods—can disrupt blood sugar regulation, promote inflammation, and drive cravings. Focus on natural sources (like fruit) and use added sugars sparingly. What matters more than grams is context: is it part of a nourishing meal, or a replacement for one?

Caffeine can enhance focus, mood, and even athletic performance in moderate amounts. Overuse, however, may interfere with sleep, increase anxiety, or cause dependence. Coffee and tea also contain antioxidants, so they aren't neutral drinks—but timing and dose matter. Be especially mindful after midday.

Alcohol deserves thoughtful consideration. While moderate consumption (like red wine) is culturally and socially integrated, emerging research suggests that even low levels may carry some health risks. That said, enjoyment and social context matter too. If you choose to drink, do so intentionally, with food, and not as a stress-reliever.

Food Synergy – How Meals Work Together

One of the most underappreciated aspects of healthy eating is not just *what* we eat, but *how* we combine foods. The concept of food synergy refers to how certain nutrients enhance each other's absorption, utilization, or effect in the body when eaten together. It shifts the focus from isolated nutrients to the bigger picture of how whole foods interact within the context of a meal.

Consider iron, an essential mineral that plays a role in oxygen transport and energy production. Non-heme iron from plant foods like lentils or spinach isn't as easily absorbed as heme iron from animal sources. But pair those lentils with vitamin C-rich foods—like a tomato salad, red peppers, or a squeeze of lemon—and you can significantly increase the iron your body absorbs. This is why cultural dishes like Indian dal with lime or Mediterranean lentil salads with chopped parsley and lemon are more than just flavorful—they're nutritionally intelligent.

Or take fat-soluble vitamins, such as A, D, E, and K. These vitamins require dietary fat to be properly absorbed. Eating a carrot, which is rich in beta-carotene (a precursor to vitamin A), alongside a fat source like olive oil, avocado, or even a few walnuts can help your body access that nutrient far more effectively. Without the fat, much of it passes through unused.

Another example is turmeric, a spice often praised for its potential anti-inflammatory properties due to a compound called curcumin. However, curcumin has low bioavailability on its own. When turmeric is consumed with black pepper (which contains piperine) and fat, absorption increases dramatically. This explains why traditional Indian cuisine often combines turmeric with ghee (a form of clarified butter) and black pepper in cooking. It's not just for taste—it's a form of nutritional wisdom passed down over generations.

Certain plant foods, when combined, can also offer a more complete protein profile. For instance, rice and beans eaten together provide all nine essential amino acids, even though each one on its own is considered "incomplete." This kind of combination is foundational in many traditional cuisines, from Latin American to Middle Eastern diets, and it reflects a deep, ancestral understanding of food synergy before science even gave it a name.

Let's also look at phytochemicals: plant compounds that may support cellular health and reduce oxidative stress. Some polyphenols found in fruits and vegetables are better absorbed when consumed with healthy fats. That means your colorful salad loaded with tomatoes, cucumbers, and leafy greens gets a major nutritional upgrade when you drizzle it with extra virgin olive oil. Or when you eat a handful of blueberries with full-fat yogurt.

Legumes and whole grains both contain phytic acid, which can bind to certain minerals and make them harder to absorb. But when these foods are soaked, sprouted, or fermented—a process used in many traditional cultures—the phytic acid decreases and mineral bioavailability improves. This is food synergy not just in the meal itself, but in how it's prepared.

Another compelling area of synergy is between fiber and fermented foods. Fiber-rich foods like oats, legumes, and vegetables serve as prebiotics, fuel for beneficial gut bacteria. Fermented foods like kefir, sauerkraut, or kimchi provide those bacteria directly (probiotics). When eaten together, these foods can create a powerful effect on gut health: the prebiotics feed the probiotics, and the result may be better digestion, immune support, and even mood regulation.

And don't overlook the value of simplicity. A well-balanced stir-fry that includes tofu (protein), broccoli (fiber and antioxidants), sesame oil (healthy fat), and brown rice (complex carbs and B vitamins) is more than a quick dinner, it's a naturally synergistic meal. The ingredients work together to support your digestion, satiety, and blood sugar stability.

When you begin to think in terms of combinations—rather than isolated foods—you move closer to the way your body actually works. It doesn't process nutrients in silos. Meals are a conversation between different ingredients, and your body listens to the whole dialogue.

So how do you apply this? You don't need a spreadsheet or a nutritional calculator. You need a few anchor principles:

- Include a source of fat with your veggies.
- Add citrus or colorful fruits when eating plant-based iron.

- Use spices generously and pair them wisely (turmeric + black pepper).
- Combine proteins strategically if you're plant-based.
- Let whole meals, not supplements, be your main source of nutrients.

Food synergy is a lens that makes meals more than just fuel. It turns your plate into a system—a dynamic, living thing that supports your energy, mood, metabolism, and more. It also helps you appreciate the wisdom behind traditional cuisines. The dishes your grandparents or ancestors made weren't just about taste or tradition—they were about balance, bioavailability, and deep nourishment, even if no one used those words.

So next time you build a meal, ask: how can I make this not just satisfying, but supportive? How can I help my body access more from less, simply by mixing ingredients with care? The answer doesn't lie in superfoods or perfection. It lies in thoughtful combinations, a little bit of knowledge, and a lot of curiosity.

Building Meals Based on Real-Life Goals

If your goal is sustained energy: Build meals with slow-digesting complex carbs like beans, oats, or sweet potatoes; include protein and healthy fats to stabilize energy over hours. Avoid starting the day with high-sugar meals or caffeine on an empty stomach.

If your goal is better focus: Include omega-3 rich foods like eggs or nuts, moderate caffeine with food, and stay well-hydrated. Avoid large, heavy meals that can drain your energy mid-day.

If your goal is better digestion: Start meals with a few deep breaths to activate your parasympathetic nervous system. Chew thoroughly. Include bitter greens and fermented foods regularly. Reduce meal size if bloating is frequent.

If your goal is mood stability: Anchor your meals with consistent eating times. Include tryptophan-rich foods (like turkey, oats, or bananas), magnesium (leafy greens, seeds), and healthy fats. Support your gut—it communicates with your brain more than we once thought.

If your goal is better sleep: Avoid late-night caffeine, heavy meals close to bedtime, and include calming foods in the evening like chamomile tea, warm broth, or a small protein snack to stabilize blood sugar overnight.

Beyond the Hype: Smart Choices in a Noisy Food World

Walk into any grocery store today and it's hard to miss the health halo effect. Products shout buzzwords like "natural," "guilt-free," "immune boosting," and "clean eating." Boxes of cereal promise digestive harmony, protein bars mimic dessert but claim to support weight loss, and the snack aisle is full of plant-based puffs and kale chips packaged to feel virtuous.

It's no wonder people are confused. Many of these products are marketed with just enough truth to sound credible—but not enough clarity to be truly helpful. The result? A fog of half-truths and healthwashing that makes eating well feel harder than it needs to be. The good news is, once you know what to look for, it's much easier to see past the hype. Real food is simple. The rest is packaging.

Food Myths That Won't Die (And What to Know Instead)

Let's unpack a few persistent myths that continue to shape buying habits:

"Agave is better than sugar."

Agave syrup is often marketed as a low-glycemic sweetener, meaning it won't spike your blood sugar as quickly as table sugar. While technically true, the full story is more complex. Agave is extremely high in fructose— a type of sugar that doesn't raise blood glucose directly but is metabolized by the liver. Excessive fructose consumption (especially in isolated form) may contribute to insulin resistance and elevated triglycerides over time.

If you're looking to sweeten something, small amounts of honey, maple syrup, or even plain sugar used sparingly are not necessarily worse. The key is frequency and quantity, not perfection. Natural doesn't always mean better.

"Gluten-free means healthy."

Unless you have celiac disease or a diagnosed gluten intolerance, gluten-free does not automatically equal healthier. In fact, many gluten-free processed foods are made with refined starches like white rice flour, tapioca starch, or potato starch—which may spike blood sugar more than their whole wheat counterparts.

Choosing gluten-free should be about your body's needs, not marketing. A gluten-free cookie is still a cookie.

"Detox teas help cleanse the body."

This idea sells a lot of tea, but the science doesn't back it. The liver and kidneys already detox your body naturally. Most so-called detox teas are simply herbal laxatives or diuretics that may lead to temporary weight loss from water and waste—not toxins.

That doesn't mean herbal teas have no value. Ginger, peppermint, or dandelion root teas can support digestion or comfort, but they aren't magic bullets. Sustainable health doesn't come from teas that promise overnight results.

"Protein bars are healthy snacks."

It depends. Many popular protein bars are candy bars in disguise: ultra-processed, high in sugar alcohols or artificial sweeteners, and often coated in chocolate or artificial flavorings. While they may be useful in a pinch or after intense training, whole food snacks like boiled eggs, nuts, or Greek yogurt typically provide more satiety with fewer additives.

A Day of Smart Eating – Case Studies in Real Life

Let's zoom out from individual ingredients and look at how a full day of eating might look when guided by the principles in this book. These aren't prescriptions—just living examples:

Case Study: Martha, 35, Freelance Designer

Goal: Stable energy, reduce afternoon crashes, eat simply without obsessing.

- **Breakfast:** Rolled oats cooked in almond milk with chia seeds, cinnamon, and frozen berries. A boiled egg on the side for protein.
- **Lunch:** Leftover roasted chicken, mixed greens, olive oil dressing, chickpeas, and roasted carrots. Water with lemon.
- **Snack:** A handful of almonds and a pear.
- **Dinner:** Stir-fried tofu with broccoli, garlic, tamari, sesame oil, served over brown rice.
- **Observation:** Meals combine fiber, fat, and protein. Blood sugar stays stable. Variety comes naturally.

Case Study: Helen, 50, Nurse on Night Shifts

Goal: Better digestion, reduce processed foods, easy prep.

- **Breakfast (post-shift):** Greek yogurt with flax seeds, banana, and walnuts.
- **Lunch (before sleeping):** Lentil soup with kale, whole grain toast with avocado.
- **Dinner (before shift):** Baked salmon, quinoa, steamed zucchini with olive oil.
- **Snack during night shift:** Homemade trail mix (pumpkin seeds, dried cherries, dark chocolate pieces).

Helen rotates simple meals, focuses on hydration, and avoids ultra-processed snacks at work. This supports his circadian rhythm without requiring extreme prep.

How to Read Labels Without Getting Duped

Here's where a lot of people feel overwhelmed. But once you learn a few principles, label-reading becomes second nature.

"Natural" means almost nothing.

In the U.S., there's no formal definition for "natural" on most food labels. It often just means the product doesn't contain artificial colors or synthetic preservatives, but it can still be heavily processed or full of sugar.

"Organic" has a defined standard, but context matters.

Organic means the product meets certain agricultural standards—free from most synthetic pesticides, non-GMO, and with animal welfare requirements. It does *not* mean the food is lower in calories, sugar, or sodium. Organic cookies are still cookies.

"Clean" is a marketing term, not a legal one.

There is no scientific or legal definition for "clean eating." What qualifies as "clean" can vary wildly between brands and influencers. Focus instead on ingredient quality and simplicity: fewer additives, fewer unpronounceables, and foods that resemble their original state.

Ingredients list: where the truth lives.

Look here first. Ingredients are listed in descending order by weight. If sugar (or its aliases like glucose, syrup, maltodextrin) is one of the first few, it's likely a sugar-heavy product no matter what the front label claims.

The Bigger Picture – Why Context Always Wins

No single ingredient, label, or trend defines your health. What matters most is the **pattern over time**. A so-called unhealthy food in the context of a balanced, mindful diet may be totally fine. A "healthy snack" eaten mindlessly or excessively doesn't become magic just because the label says so.Food is more than fuel. It's culture, comfort, and connection. It's also chemistry, and that's where food synergy, nutrient absorption, and meal composition come into play. What works for your friend might not be right for you. Your life, your preferences, your body's feedback—those are your best guides. Use knowledge as a compass, not a cage.

Health Across the Seasons of Life

One of the most liberating truths about health is that it doesn't require perfection—it requires adaptability. Our needs evolve. Our energy shifts. Life hands us different responsibilities, opportunities, and stressors at different stages. But what doesn't change is our ability to respond with awareness, self-respect, and small, meaningful choices.

This chapter isn't about age-based rules. It's about recognizing how the same health foundation: real food, rest, movement, emotional clarity, can be applied differently as we grow. Because sustainable health isn't just about what you do. It's about *how* you do it, and when.

Your 20s to 30s – Building the Base

This is often a phase of high energy, but also high distraction. Many people in this season are building careers, navigating social identity, or adjusting to independence. Health may not always feel urgent—but this is where your baseline is formed.

Metabolism is typically more forgiving, but that doesn't mean it's invincible. Over-reliance on caffeine, erratic eating patterns, or sleep deprivation may not feel serious now, but they plant seeds that show up later. The good news? This is an ideal window for building default habits that carry you into the next chapters with less effort.

If you're in this season:

- Practice cooking simple meals. You don't need to be a chef—just confident with a skillet and a grocery list.
- Prioritize sleep even if no one else around you is. Late nights feel fun until they're routine.
- Exercise for strength and mobility, not just aesthetics. What you build now becomes your reserve later.

- Watch your self-talk. Body image can be noisy in this decade. Learning to respect your body instead of fight it creates resilience that no diet can deliver.

This isn't about pressure to get everything perfect. It's about planting habits you'll be glad to have when things get more complex.

Your 40s to 50s – Adapting to Change

This phase often comes with major shifts—physically, hormonally, and emotionally. You may notice your recovery time changing. Sleep may feel different. Weight might shift even though your habits haven't. Hormonal transitions (especially for women) can impact energy, mood, and metabolism. This isn't failure. It's biology. And it's an invitation to adjust, not give up.

What may support you now:

- Strength training becomes a priority, not a luxury. Muscle mass naturally declines with age, but lifting weights (even bodyweight) can help preserve it.
- Sleep quality matters more than ever. If it's disrupted, focus on light exposure, wind-down routines, and reducing stimulants.
- Blood sugar sensitivity may increase. Balanced meals with fiber, protein, and fat can help stabilize energy.
- Emotional health matters deeply. Many people in this phase face caregiving demands, work stress, or identity shifts. Tools like journaling, therapy, or mindfulness may be as essential as nutrition.

Adapting isn't about doing less. It's about doing what fits *now* with clarity and self-respect.

Your 60s and Beyond – Gentle Resilience

Later decades of life are often painted with extremes: either hyper-vigilant health regimens or total neglect. But there's a softer, more empowering approach: gentle resilience. At this stage, the goal isn't optimization—it's maintenance, enjoyment, and quality of life.

Mobility and balance become top priorities. These are the foundations for independence and confidence. Whether it's yoga, walking, swimming, or tai chi, consistent movement helps maintain strength and reduce fall risk.

Nutritional needs shift too. Protein becomes more important to help maintain muscle. Appetite might change, so nutrient-dense foods in smaller portions can help. Hydration is sometimes overlooked but remains crucial. Mental and emotional health often become clearer priorities. Social connection, purpose, and creativity may provide more energy than any supplement. If you're in this season:

- Keep meals simple, colorful, and easy to digest.
- Use movement as a form of self-respect, not punishment.
- Prioritize meaningful routines and relationships.
- Remember: it's never too late. Small changes still matter.

This phase isn't a decline—it's a recalibration. What you do now can still nourish your future.

Across All Ages – What Never Changes

No matter where you are in life, some things are always the same and some truths remain:

Sleep matters, always. Whether you're 25 or 75, restorative sleep supports every system in your body. The way you get there might change, but the need doesn't.

Real food still wins. Fads come and go. What stays consistent is the power of whole, minimally processed foods: fruits, vegetables, proteins, fats, legumes, and grains.

Stress management isn't optional. Whether it's exams, parenting, retirement transitions, or health diagnoses: the ability to self-regulate matters. Stress has a huge impact on our health.

Movement is medicine. There is no age where walking, stretching, or lifting stops being beneficial. It just looks different over time.

Flexibility wins over rigidity. Life changes. Schedules change. Energy changes. Your habits need to flex with you—not bind you.

Kindness matters most. Judgment never builds consistency. Compassion does. The longer your journey, the more this truth shows up.

A Final Reminder

No matter what decade you're in, your health isn't behind. There is no ideal timeline. What you do next is always more important than what you didn't do yesterday. You don't have to become someone new. You just have to keep listening, adjusting, and staying present. That's what health actually is: attention, action, and adaptability over time. In our final chapter, we'll talk about how to think clearly in a world that constantly sells confusion—and how to trust yourself more deeply along the way.

How to Think Critically in a Confusing Wellness World

We live in a time when you can access more health information in a single afternoon than your grandparents could in a lifetime. And yet, despite this abundance, clarity remains elusive. Contradictory headlines, influencer advice, miracle supplements, fear-based warnings—it's easy to feel overwhelmed or even paralyzed.

That's why this final chapter exists: not to give you more rules, but to hand you a filter. A way to sort truth from noise. A framework to help you keep your feet on the ground in a wellness world that often feels like quicksand. When you can think clearly, you can act confidently. That doesn't mean you need to become a scientist. It means learning how to ask good questions, recognize red flags, and stay curious without getting swept up in hype.

What "Evidence-Based" Really Means

You'll hear the phrase "evidence-based" a lot in the health world, often as a badge of credibility. But not all evidence is equal, and not all uses of the word are honest.

In science, evidence exists on a spectrum. At the bottom is anecdotal evidence: individual stories or personal results. These can be valuable, but they're not enough to make broad recommendations. Your neighbor might swear by a juice cleanse, but that doesn't mean it's universally helpful.

Higher up the ladder are observational studies, which look for patterns in large groups of people. These can suggest associations (like high vegetable intake and lower risk of disease), but they don't prove cause and effect. The gold standard? Randomized controlled trials (RCTs), where groups are randomly assigned an intervention or a placebo. These can help show whether a treatment or habit has a measurable impact.

Even higher are meta-analyses, which combine multiple RCTs to detect larger patterns.

Still, even strong evidence doesn't mean a recommendation is right *for you*. Research can tell us what tends to work on average. It can't always predict how an individual body will respond. That's where personal awareness comes in—and why your lived experience matters alongside science.

Red Flags in Wellness Marketing

If you've ever been targeted by an ad for a "belly fat torching" tea or "total body reset" supplement, you already know how persuasive wellness marketing can be. It's often designed to trigger urgency, shame, or FOMO (fear of missing out). Here's what to look out for:

- **Too-good-to-be-true promises.** Claims like "lose 10 pounds in a week" or "never get sick again" are red flags. Health doesn't work in absolutes.
- **Fear-based messaging.** Warnings about "toxins," "chemicals," or "poisonous" ingredients are often exaggerated without context.
- **Testimonials over science.** Stories are powerful, but they're not proof. One person's result does not guarantee yours.
- **Use of "natural" as a halo.** Natural doesn't always mean safe. Arsenic is natural. So is poison ivy. Effectiveness depends on evidence, not origin.
- **Scientific jargon with no clarity.** If a product says it "supports detox pathways via mitochondrial modulation," and there's no clear explanation or citation, be cautious.

The goal isn't to reject everything. It's to develop a healthy skepticism. Ask: Who benefits if I believe this? Where is the source? Is there independent evidence?

How to Ask Better Questions

Curiosity is your best defense against confusion. When you hear a new health claim, try these internal prompts:

- **What problem is this trying to solve?** Does that problem even apply to me?
- **Where did this advice come from?** Is it peer-reviewed research, or an influencer with a promo code?
- **Does it align with basic principles?** If it contradicts everything you know about sleep, food, or movement, question it.
- **What does my body say?** If you've tried something new, what happened? Did you feel better, worse, the same?

Example: You read about intermittent fasting. Before jumping in, you could ask: Does skipping breakfast feel sustainable for me? What does the research actually say about benefits and limitations? How does it impact energy, stress, or mood in my real life?

This doesn't mean second-guessing yourself into paralysis. It means creating a habit of thoughtful curiosity. Not because you don't trust anyone—but because your health is worth thinking deeply about.

When to Consult a Professional

Critical thinking includes knowing your limits. There are times when self-education isn't enough, and getting help from a professional is the smartest move you can make.

Here's when you might consider it:

- Persistent fatigue, pain, or digestion issues that don't improve.
- Concerns about medication, supplements, or chronic symptoms.
- Major life changes: pregnancy, menopause, surgery recovery.
- Mental health struggles like anxiety, depression, or burnout.

The key is finding a provider who listens, collaborates, and respects your autonomy. Not all practitioners are equal—but many are thoughtful allies who can help you interpret your experience through a clinical lens.

If you're unsure where to start:

- Ask for recommendations from people you trust.
- Look for credentials like RDN (Registered Dietitian Nutritionist), MD (Medical Doctor), or licensed therapists.
- Don't be afraid to ask a provider how they make recommendations. A good one won't be offended—they'll welcome the conversation.

Building Trust in Yourself

The ultimate goal of this chapter isn't to make you skeptical of everything. It's to help you become a more grounded, empowered consumer of health information. You don't need to know every answer. But you do need to trust your ability to pause, think, and choose based on values rather than panic. Health doesn't live in extremes. It thrives in nuance. That's why critical thinking isn't about saying no to everything. It's about knowing when to say yes—and being confident in why.

In our final pages, we'll offer a gentle send-off. Not a summary or recap, but a reflection. Because while *health* may be simple, *you* are complex—and that's a beautiful thing to honor.

The Minimalist Health Mindset

We live in an age of excess — not of food or possessions alone, but of *inputs*. Every minute, our senses, devices, and thoughts compete for attention. Notifications flash, opinions multiply, and expectations pile up. Even our health journeys, meant to simplify and restore, often become tangled in advice, gadgets, and goals. The result is paradoxical: we are surrounded by abundance yet starving for peace.

The minimalist health mindset begins where overload ends. It's not about having less — it's about *needing less to feel whole*. It's a mindset that redefines success not as doing everything, but as doing what truly matters. It's the natural continuation of everything this book has been building toward: understanding health not as another project to manage, but as a way of being that honors simplicity, space, and focus.

The Weight of Overstimulation

The modern nervous system is doing something it was never designed to do: process thousands of pieces of information per day. Our ancestors navigated a sensory world of patterns, light, sound, and immediate experiences — wind, voices, the rustle of animals. Today, the mind is bombarded with messages, alerts, marketing, and screens. The eyes never rest. The mind never idles. And the cost is measurable.

Chronic stimulation keeps the body in a subtle state of vigilance. Cortisol and adrenaline, meant to rise briefly in response to threat, become constant background noise. The attention system, built to focus on one meaningful task, gets fragmented. Over time, overstimulation leads to fatigue, irritability, insomnia, and anxiety — symptoms we often blame on diet or workload, when the real culprit is overload itself.

Information overload is not just mental — it's *metabolic*. Every bit of sensory input requires energy to process. Studies in cognitive neuroscience show that the prefrontal cortex — the brain region responsible for decision-making and focus — tires with excess stimulation, leading to reduced willpower and poor emotional regulation. The mind becomes cluttered, and so does behavior: multitasking replaces mindfulness, reaction replaces reflection.

The body follows. When mental space is crowded, sleep suffers, digestion slows, and inflammation rises. The nervous system has no "off switch" when stimulation is constant. It's as though the light of consciousness burns continuously, with no night to recover. The minimalist health mindset begins by recognizing that rest, clarity, and focus are not luxuries — they are biological necessities.

The Myth of More

Somewhere along the way, society began equating *more* with *better.* More productivity meant more success. More data meant more control. More supplements meant more health. But the truth is that excess creates noise — and noise is the enemy of balance.

In health culture especially, the "more" trap is everywhere. One more diet, one more tracker, one more superfood. We're encouraged to micromanage our bodies as though complexity guarantees control. Yet every extra rule, gadget, and piece of advice adds cognitive load. We end up juggling ideas instead of listening to the body.

Minimalism is a counterculture to this mindset. It doesn't reject progress; it filters it. It asks: *what truly adds value to my life, and what just adds friction?* In the same way your body filters toxins, your mind must filter attention. Every unnecessary input is a kind of mental waste — clutter that consumes energy and attention that could be used for healing.

When you adopt minimalism in health, you stop chasing the perfect system and start practicing discernment. You learn to distinguish between what helps and what merely distracts. You realize that wellbeing grows not by accumulation, but by subtraction.

117

Mental and Emotional Decluttering

The mind, like a home, gathers clutter. Not just thoughts, but unprocessed worries, self-criticism, comparisons, and plans. Over time, that clutter fills every mental corner, leaving no space for calm. Mental minimalism begins with awareness. It's the quiet recognition that you don't have to think about everything all the time. The mind's job isn't to hold every thought — it's to process what's relevant and let the rest pass through. Most of us were never taught to let thoughts go. We collect them, turn them over, and replay them endlessly. That repetition drains the same energy we need for focus and joy.

Emotional minimalism extends this idea to feelings. It doesn't mean repressing emotion; it means simplifying how we respond to it. You can feel sadness without adding a story about failure. You can feel stress without layering guilt on top. Emotions are signals, not verdicts. Minimalism in emotion is learning to experience them cleanly — to let a wave rise and fall without building a storm around it.

One practical exercise: at the end of each day, ask yourself, *"What truly mattered today?"* Write one or two sentences — not tasks, but moments or insights that carried meaning. Over time, you'll notice that very few things actually define your days. This reflection naturally trims the mental clutter that doesn't serve your health. When the mind quiets, the body follows. Breath deepens. The heart rate steadies. Sleep improves. It's not magic — it's physiology responding to simplicity.

The Power of Empty Space

In architecture, empty space gives form to a room. In music, silence gives meaning to sound. In life, stillness gives context to action. But in our culture, stillness often feels wasteful. Doing nothing is seen as unproductive, even shameful. We fill every gap — with screens, noise, or multitasking — until the absence of input feels uncomfortable.

Yet those empty moments are where recovery happens. The parasympathetic nervous system activates only when the mind stops striving. It's in pauses — the walk without headphones, the meal without a podcast, the morning without instant scrolling — that the body recalibrates. Minimalism teaches us to value that emptiness. Not as a void to be filled, but as space to be inhabited. Health doesn't come from constant doing; it comes from alternating effort with rest, stimulation with silence. Without those cycles, we burn out. Try reclaiming small spaces of nothingness throughout your day: five minutes of breathing before you reach for your phone, a quiet moment after meals, or a short walk without distractions. These pauses are not luxuries — they're maintenance for the mind.

Simplifying Routines and Commitments

When every day feels rushed, even healthy habits become chores. The minimalist health mindset reframes routines as *anchors*, not obligations. Instead of chasing the perfect morning routine, it asks: *What few habits consistently make me feel grounded?* Maybe it's a short stretch, a balanced breakfast, or a few minutes of journaling. Choose the minimum effective dose — the small, sustainable core that keeps you steady.

The same applies to commitments. Many people stay in a state of perpetual overwhelm because they say yes out of guilt or habit. But every "yes" is a withdrawal of energy from something else. Minimalism requires the courage to say no — not from selfishness, but from clarity. You can't restore your body if your schedule is permanently full. Your nervous system needs blank spaces as much as your calendar does. Ask yourself regularly: *If I stopped doing this, what would really happen?* You'll find that much of what consumes your time adds little to your health or purpose. Simplifying commitments isn't about isolation; it's about making room for depth — for the few things and people that truly matter.

Decluttering the Environment

Our surroundings constantly speak to the nervous system. A cluttered room, overflowing inbox, or messy desk sends signals of unfinished business. The body interprets that as mild tension, even if you don't consciously notice it.

Environmental minimalism is about aligning your space with your biology. Start small: clear one surface, one drawer, one corner. Don't think in terms of perfection; think in terms of calm. When visual noise decreases, the mind naturally focuses. Studies show that clean, organized spaces reduce cortisol and improve concentration. The brain prefers order — not for aesthetic reasons, but because order signals safety.

Minimalism at home also means designing spaces that invite rest. Keep your sleep area screen-free. Use warm, dim lighting in the evening. Keep objects visible only if they serve or soothe you. These small choices reinforce physiological calm every day, without requiring willpower. As your environment quiets, internal noise follows. You start to feel a subtle spaciousness — not just in your room, but in your mind.

Digital Hygiene: Reclaiming Attention

If there's one domain where minimalism is most needed, it's the digital world.

Our attention has become the most valuable currency on Earth — traded, tracked, and monetized. Every notification, vibration, or suggestion is engineered to steal a second of focus. The result is fragmented awareness and a nervous system in constant alert. Digital hygiene is the modern form of self-protection. It doesn't require abandoning technology — it means using it deliberately.

Here are guiding principles (not a list of rules, but attitudes):

- **Boundaries of time:** Designate screen-free zones — the first 30 minutes after waking and the last 30 before bed are ideal. These are the windows when your subconscious is most open. Protect them from external noise.

- **Boundaries of purpose:** Before opening a device, ask, *"What am I here for?"* Enter with intention, not reflex.
- **Boundaries of space:** Keep devices out of sight during meals and rest. The simple act of putting the phone in another room can restore attention more effectively than any app.
- **Boundaries of input:** Curate what you consume. Unfollow sources that spark anxiety or comparison. Subscribe only to voices that educate, uplift, or calm.

You don't have to delete everything. Just reduce the noise until what remains supports who you want to become. Minimalist digital living is not deprivation — it's liberation. It reclaims your most precious resource: *presence.*

Restoring Depth in a Shallow World

Depth takes time, and time has become scarce. When life is lived in notifications and quick reactions, deep focus and real relationships fade. The minimalist health mindset invites you to reverse that trend. Spend more time doing fewer things. Read one book slowly instead of ten summaries. Have one meaningful conversation instead of dozens of half-thought exchanges. Cook one nourishing meal instead of juggling multiple health hacks. Depth multiplies satisfaction. It slows the nervous system and restores the sense of coherence that overstimulation erodes.

Minimalism reminds us that health is not intensity; it's consistency. The same way a plant doesn't thrive under constant watering but steady care, your well-being depends on sustainable rhythms. You don't need constant novelty — you need space for growth.

The Minimalist Body: Doing Less, Healing More

In fitness culture, rest is often underrated. Yet growth happens not during exertion but during recovery. The same principle applies to all aspects of health. When you stop overwhelming your system with inputs — dietary, sensory, emotional — the body uses that freed energy for repair.

Minimalism in movement means training intelligently, not endlessly. It's taking a walk instead of forcing a workout when exhausted. It's trusting that balance creates progress faster than punishment. Minimalism in nutrition means focusing on whole, unprocessed foods, not chasing perfection. It's understanding that eating simply and consistently is more healing than obsessing over micronutrient data. Minimalism is physiological efficiency — doing enough to trigger adaptation, then allowing the system to restore. The body loves rhythm, not excess. When you give it space, it recalibrates toward equilibrium.

The Calm Mind as a Biological Advantage

A minimalist mind is a focused mind, and focus changes physiology. Brain imaging studies show that mindfulness and attention control reduce activity in the amygdala (the fear center) and increase activation in the prefrontal cortex (the center of rational control and compassion). This leads to lower blood pressure, improved digestion, and better immune response. When attention is scattered, the brain operates in constant threat mode. When attention is directed, the body shifts to healing. In that sense, minimalism isn't philosophical — it's neurological. It's training your mind to stop multitasking and start inhabiting the present moment fully.

You can practice this anytime: washing dishes, breathing between tasks, or even walking. Do one thing, feel it completely, then move on. Each single-task moment strengthens the neural circuits of calm. The more you practice, the easier it becomes to sustain clarity amid chaos.

Minimalism as Empowerment, Not Restriction

Many people mistake minimalism for deprivation — as though reducing stimuli means reducing joy. In reality, minimalism expands joy. It's the difference between noise and music. By clearing what's meaningless, you make room for what moves you deeply.

When you no longer chase every new idea or product, you rediscover gratitude for what you already have. Meals taste better. Rest feels more restorative. Relationships gain texture. The mind, no longer divided, can finally experience the richness that simplicity reveals. Minimalism is not a rule: it's a lens. It helps you ask, again and again: *Is this helping me live more fully?* If not, it can go.

A Quiet Finish

By now, you've read many pages. You've thought through food, movement, sleep, mindset, emotions, toxins, habits, and health misinformation. You've explored both the scientific side of wellness and the deeply personal experience of living in a human body. But this last chapter isn't here to summarize what you already know. You don't need a recap—you need space. Space to step back, breathe, and look at your life with the eyes of someone who now sees health not as a project, but as a pattern.

Let this final stretch be less about conclusions and more about anchoring. You didn't come here for a formula. You came for clarity. So let's end with that.

Simplicity Is Not the Same as Laziness

We live in a culture that often confuses intensity with intelligence. If a plan isn't extreme, it must not be effective. If a person isn't "all in," they must not care. Simplicity, in this kind of world, gets dismissed as basic, boring, or uninformed. But let's be clear: simplicity is not laziness. Simplicity is what remains when you strip away the noise and keep what works. Anyone can build a complicated wellness routine. But it takes real maturity to ask: what's actually helping me? What can I stop pretending to need? You may have noticed this in your own life: that the most powerful shifts weren't the loudest ones. Maybe it was going to bed an hour earlier. Or eating breakfast for the first time in years. Or deciding to walk every evening instead of chasing the perfect workout.

Making Peace with Progress

One of the hardest things in any health journey is letting go of the fantasy version of yourself. The one who wakes up at 5am, meal preps like a pro, never eats late, and somehow glows with natural discipline.

That version might sell on Instagram. But it's not the person who does the grocery shopping when you're exhausted or gently stretches before bed when the day's been hard.

Progress, in real life, is uneven. You will forget things. You will go through seasons where everything feels off. That's not failure, that's rhythm. What matters isn't whether you stayed "on track." What matters is whether you kept returning to yourself. To your body. To your truth. That's what makes this sustainable.

You Don't Have to Earn Your Health

So many of us grew up with the idea that health is something we must deserve. That we have to be thin enough, clean enough, disciplined enough to qualify. That wellness is a badge we earn through self-denial.

But your body is not a battleground. It's not a machine to optimize or a problem to fix. It's a living, breathing companion. A collaborator. Something to partner with, not dominate. You don't have to earn the right to feel good. You don't have to hit a certain weight or cleanse your kitchen or eliminate every indulgence. You are allowed to care for yourself simply because you exist. Health is not a prize, it's a practice. One that honors your biology, your story, and your circumstances.

What You Carry Forward

If this book has done its job, you're leaving not with a list of rules, but with a new lens. A way of seeing your body and your habits not as chores, but as acts of respect. You carry forward the knowledge that real food works, even when trends shift. That sleep matters, even when hustle is glamorized. That movement is your birthright, not a punishment. That emotions and stress affect your health just as deeply as any vitamin.

But most of all, you carry the ability to ask better questions.

Questions like:

- What does my body need today, not just what should I do?
- Am I acting out of curiosity or fear?
- What would this look like if it were easy?

These questions guide you when things get noisy again—because they will. Life will throw new obligations, conflicting advice, and changing circumstances. But the quiet confidence you've built? That stays.

The Courage to Be Gentle

It takes courage to be gentle in a world that rewards extremes. To choose small, consistent change instead of chasing dramatic results. To eat nourishing food without turning it into obsession. To move because it feels good, not because you're punishing yourself. Gentleness isn't weakness. It's wisdom. It's what allows you to stay in the game when others burn out. It's what lets you enjoy the process instead of waiting for the perfect moment. Let your health be a relationship, not a project. Something that unfolds, evolves, and adjusts with you.

From Here On

There is no perfect plan to follow next. There is no 30-day program waiting in the appendix. There is just you.

You, in your kitchen. You, on your walk. You, lying awake at night deciding whether to reach for your phone or take a breath. You, at the grocery store. You, when things fall apart. You, when they come back together. You already know more than you think. You've lived in this body your whole life. The tools are here. The rest is practice. This book ends. But your life's rhythm continues. And with it, your chance to return—again and again—to what's real.

Because real health isn't about being perfect all the time,
It's about being present and consistent.
And that, more than anything, is simple.

Thank you for reading these pages.
May your next meal be peaceful, your next breath intentional, and your next choice one that brings you closer to yourself.

www.ingramcontent.com/pod-product-compliance
Lightning Source LLC
Chambersburg PA
CBHW052137270326
41930CB00012B/2928